New Advances in Hepatic Encephalopathy

Editor

ROBERT S. BROWN Jr

CLINICS IN LIVER DISEASE

www.liver.theclinics.com

Consulting Editor
NORMAN GITLIN

August 2015 • Volume 19 • Number 3

ELSEVIER

1600 John F. Kennedy Boulevard • Suite 1800 • Philadelphia, Pennsylvania, 19103-2899

http://www.theclinics.com

CLINICS IN LIVER DISEASE Volume 19, Number 3
August 2015 ISSN 1089-3261, ISBN-13: 978-0-323-37603-7

Editor: Kerry Holland
Developmental Editor: Meredith Clinton

Clinics in Liver Disease (ISSN 1089-3261) is published quarterly by Elsevier Inc., 360 Park Avenue South, New York, NY 10010-1710. Months of issue are February, May, August, and November. Business and Editorial Offices: 1600 John F. Kennedy Blvd., Ste. 1800, Philadelphia, PA 19103-2899. Customer Service Office: 3251 Riverport Lane, Maryland Heights, MO 63043. Periodicals postage paid at New York, NY and additional mailing offices. Subscription prices are $295.00 per year (U.S. individuals), $145.00 per year (U.S. student/resident), $401.00 per year (U.S. institutions), $395.00 per year (international individuals), $200.00 per year (international student/resident), $498.00 per year (international instituitions), $340.00 per year (Canadian individuals), $200.00 per year (Canadian student/resident), and $498.00 per year (Canadian institutions). Foreign air speed delivery is included in all Clinics subscription prices. All prices are subject to change without notice. **POSTMASTER:** Send address changes to Clinics in Liver Disease, Elsevier Health Sciences Division, Subscription Customer Service, 3251 Riverport Lane, Maryland Heights, MO 63043. **Customer Service: Telephone: 1-800-654-2452 (U.S. and Canada); 314-447-8871 (outside U.S. and Canada). Fax: 314-447-8029. E-mail: journalscustomer service-usa@elsevier.com (for print support); journalsonlinesupport-usa@elsevier.com (for online support).**

Reprints. For copies of 100 or more of articles in this publication, please contact the Commercial Reprints Department, Elsevier Inc., 360 Park Avenue South, New York, NY 10010-1710. Tel.: 212-633-3874; Fax: 212-633-3820; E-mail: reprints@elsevier.com.

Clinics in Liver Disease is covered in MEDLINE/PubMed (Index Medicus), Science Citation Index Expanded, Journal Citation Reports/Science Edition, and Current Contents/Clinical Medicine.

Contributors

CONSULTING EDITOR

NORMAN GITLIN, MD, FRCP (LONDON), FRCPE (EDINBURGH), FAASLD, FACP, FACG
Formerly, Professor of Medicine, Chief of Hepatology, Emory University; Currently,
Consultant, Atlanta Gastroenterology Associates, Atlanta, Georgia

EDITOR

ROBERT S. BROWN Jr, MD, MPH
Vice Chair, Transitions of Care; Interim Chief, Division of Gastroenterology and
Hepatology, Weill Cornell Medical College, New York, New York

AUTHORS

GEORGE G. ABDELSAYED, MD, FACP, FACG
Director, Division of Gastroenterology and Hepatology, Staten Island University Hospital,
Staten Island, New York

LUIS A. BALART, MD, MACG
Chief, Division of Gastroenterology and Hepatology; Professor of Medicine, Department of
Internal Medicine, Tulane University, New Orleans, Louisiana

P. PATRICK BASU, MD, MRCP, AGAF, FACG
Assistant Clinical Professor of Medicine, Department of Medicine, Columbia University
College of Physicians and Surgeons, New York, New York; Director of Liver and Clinical
Liver Research, Department of Medicine, King's County Hospital Medical Center,
Brooklyn, New York

RAJA G.R. EDULA, MD, MRCP (UK)
Division of Gastroenterology and Hepatology, Rutgers New Jersey Medical School,
Newark, New Jersey

STEVEN L. FLAMM, MD
Professor of Medicine; Chief, Liver Transplantation Program, Northwestern Feinberg
School of Medicine, Chicago, Illinois

PHILLIP K. HENDERSON, DO
Clinical Instructor, Division of Gastroenterology, University of South Alabama, Mobile,
Alabama

JORGE L. HERRERA, MD
Professor of Medicine; Director, Division of Hepatology, University of South Alabama,
Mobile, Alabama

SUDHA KODALI, MD
Department of Gastroenterology and Hepatology, University of Alabama at Birmingham,
Birmingham, Alabama

CATHERINE LUCERO, MD
Division of Digestive and Liver Diseases, Department of Medicine, Center for Liver Disease and Transplantation, Columbia University College of Physicians and Surgeons, New York, New York

BRENDAN M. McGUIRE, MD
Department of Gastroenterology and Hepatology, University of Alabama at Birmingham, Birmingham, Alabama

PARTH J. PAREKH, MD
Division of Gastroenterology and Hepatology, Department of Internal Medicine, Tulane University, New Orleans, Louisiana

NIKOLAOS T. PYRSOPOULOS, MD, PhD, MBA
Division of Gastroenterology and Hepatology, Rutgers New Jersey Medical School, Newark, New Jersey

ROBERT S. RAHIMI, MD, MS
Annette C. and Harold C. Simmons Transplant Institute, Baylor University Medical Center; Assistant Professor, Department of Internal Medicine, Texas A&M Health Science Center, College of Medicine, Dallas, Texas

DON C. ROCKEY, MD
Professor and Chairman, Department of Internal Medicine, Medical University of South Carolina, Charleston, South Carolina

NIRAJ JAMES SHAH, MD
Internal Medicine Resident, Department of Medicine, James J. Peters VA Medical Center, Icahn School of Medicine at Mount Sinai, New York, New York

NORMAN L. SUSSMAN, MD, FAASLD
Associate Professor of Surgery, Baylor College of Medicine and Baylor-St. Luke's Medical Center, Division of Abdominal Transplantation, Houston, Texas

ELIZABETH C. VERNA, MD, MS
Assistant Professor of Medicine, Division of Digestive and Liver Diseases, Department of Medicine, Center for Liver Disease and Transplantation, Columbia University College of Physicians and Surgeons, New York, New York

JOHN M. VIERLING, MD, FACP, FAASLD
Professor of Medicine and Surgery; Chief of Hepatology; Director of Baylor Liver Health; Director of Advanced Liver Therapies, Baylor St. Luke's Liver Center, Baylor College of Medicine, Houston, Texas

Contents

> The diagnosis of hepatic encephalopathy is predominantly clinical, and the tests available assist in the diagnosis only by excluding other causes. Covert hepatic encephalopathy, which is defined as abnormal performance on psychometric tests when standard neurologic examination is completely normal, has gained widespread attention in recent years due to its effect on quality of life. This review focuses on the tests available to aid in the diagnosis of this significant complication of liver disease, and discusses the complex pathophysiologic mechanisms identified through new imaging techniques and their significance toward development of new therapeutic targets for this condition.

> Hepatic encephalopathy (HE) shows a wide spectrum of neuropsychiatric manifestations. A combined effort with neuropsychological and psychometric evaluation has to be performed to recognize the syndrome, whereas minimal HE (MHE) is largely under-recognized. Subtle symptoms of MHE can only be diagnosed through specialized neuropsychiatric testing. Early diagnosis and treatment may drastically improve the quality of life for many cirrhotic patients. Further research to gain better insight into the pathophysiology and diagnostic accuracy of HE will help determine future management strategies.

> Covert hepatic encephalopathy is a common problem in cirrhosis, affecting up to 80% of patients. It is defined as test-dependent brain dysfunction with clinical consequences in the setting of cirrhosis in patients who are not disoriented. Because it is not apparent clinically, and diagnostic testing has not been standardized, the issue has often been ignored in clinical practice. Yet, the clinical consequences are notable, including impaired quality of life, diminished work productivity, and poor driving skills.

> Hepatic encephalopathy exists along a continuum from abnormal neuropsychiatric testing in the absence of clinical findings to varying

degrees of detectable clinical findings. The International Society for Hepatic Encephalopathy and Nitrogen Metabolism has endorsed the term "covert" to encompass minimal hepatic encephalopathy and grade I overt hepatic encephalopathy. Covert hepatic encephalopathy has been associated with poor quality of life, decreased employment, increased falls, and increased traffic accidents that significantly impact quality of life and health care expenditures. Probiotics, nonabsorbable dissacharides, rifaximin, and L-ornithine-L-aspartate have been evaluated with varying levels of success. Because of the lack of universally accepted diagnostic tools, optimal timing of testing and treatment remains controversial.

As many as 80% of patients with end-stage liver disease and hepatic encephalopathy have significant protein-calorie malnutrition. Because of the severe hypercatabolic state of cirrhosis, the provision of liberal amounts of carbohydrate (at least 35 to 40 kcal/kg per day), and between 1.2 and 1.6 g/kg of protein is necessary. Protein restriction is not recommended. Branched-chain amino acid supplementation and vegetable protein are associated with improved outcomes. Dietary supplementation with vitamins, minerals (with the notable exception of zinc) and probiotics should be decided on a case-by-case basis.

Normal regulation of total body and circulating ammonia requires a delicate interplay in ammonia formation and breakdown between several organ systems. In the setting of cirrhosis and portal hypertension, the decreased hepatic clearance of ammonia leads to significant dependence on skeletal muscle for ammonia detoxification; however, cirrhosis is also associated with muscle depletion and decreased functional muscle mass. Thus, patients with diminished muscle mass and sarcopenia may have a decreased ability to compensate for hepatic insufficiency and a higher likelihood of developing physiologically significant hyperammonemia and hepatic encephalopathy.

Hepatic encephalopathy (HE) is a commonly encountered sequela of chronic liver disease and cirrhosis with significant associated morbidity and mortality. Although ammonia is implicated in the pathogenesis of HE, the exact underlying mechanisms still remain poorly understood. Its role in the urea cycle, astrocyte swelling, and glutamine and gamma-amino-n-butyric acid systems suggests that the pathogenesis is multifaceted. Greater understanding in its underlying mechanism may offer more targeted therapeutic options in the future, and thus further research is necessary to fully understand the pathogenesis of HE.

Hepatic encephalopathy (HE) is a common complication of cirrhosis, leading to frequent hospitalizations. Because ammonia is thought to play an important role in the pathogenesis of HE, therapies specifically aimed at reducing ammonia levels have been developed for conditions causing hyperammonemia, including HE. Ammonia scavengers have been used in HE patients, leading to improvements in symptoms. Bowel cleansing with polyethylene glycol has also been studied recently, resulting in more rapid improvement in acute HE compared with lactulose. Extracorporeal devices have been used in cases of refractory HE but currently are used primarily in research settings and not approved for clinical management for HE.

Hepatic encephalopathy (HE) is defined by an altered mental status in the setting of portosystemic shunting, with or without cirrhosis. The basis of HE is probably multi-factorial, but increased ammonia delivery to the brain is thought to play a pivotal role. Medical therapies have typically focused on reducing blood ammonia concentrations. These measures are moderately effective, but further improvements will require identification of new therapeutic targets. Two medications, lactulose and rifaximin, are currently approved for the treatment of HE in the USA - new compounds are available off-label, and are in clinical trials. The presence of HE is associated with a higher risk of death in cirrhotic patients. Liver transplantation typically cures HE, but HE does not increase the MELD score, and therefore does not contribute to the likelihood of liver transplantation.

Hepatic encephalopathy (HE) is associated with cerebral edema (CE), increased intracranial pressure (ICP), and subsequent neurologic complications; it is the most important cause of morbidity and mortality in fulminant hepatic failure. The goal of therapy should be early diagnosis and treatment of HE with measures to reduce CE. A combination of clinical examination and diagnostic modalities can aid in prompt diagnosis. ICP monitoring and transcranial Doppler help diagnose and monitor response to treatment. Transfer to a transplant center and intensive care unit admission with airway management and reduction of CE with hypertonic saline, mannitol, hypothermia, and sedation are recommended as a bridge to liver transplantation.

Both covert hepatic encephalopathy (CHE) and overt hepatic encephalopathy (OHE) impair the ability to operate machinery. The legal responsibilities of US physicians who diagnose and treat patients with hepatic encephalopathy vary among states. It is imperative that physicians know the laws regarding reporting in their state. OHE represents a neuropsychiatric impairment that meets general reporting criteria. The medical advisory boards of the states have not identified OHE as a reportable condition. In the absence of validated diagnostic guidelines, physicians are not obligated to perform tests for CHE. There is a need for explicit guidance from professional associations regarding this issue.

CLINICS IN LIVER DISEASE

Preface

HE or not HE? That is Frequently the Question

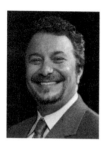

Robert S. Brown Jr, MD, MPH
Editor

Hepatic encephalopathy (HE) is a frequent clinical challenge for gastroenterologists in that the diagnosis is often unclear and the approved therapies are often inadequate and may have side effects that affect compliance. Clearly, HE has a negative impact on the patient's quality of life and that of their caregivers. In this issue of *Clinics in Liver Disease*, our authors provide a comprehensive update of the newest data in HE with a focus on diagnostics, therapeutics, and the clinical implications of HE for our patients. We start with new methods of testing and brain imaging: Drs Edula, Nikolaos, and Pyrsopoulos review new and innovative ways to make diagnoses of HE, which is critical particularly in the early or covert phases. It has also been unclear what to do when we find covert or minimal encephalopathy. Drs Basu and Shah review the clinical and neurologic manifestations of covert HE, and the treatment options are reviewed by Dr Flamm and Drs Henderson and Herrera, including the controversy as to whether this should be treated.

Dietary restriction has been a controversial area in HE; protein restriction, which used to be the standard, has clearly been debunked as a treatment modality as discussed in Dr Abdelsayed's article on nutrition and HE. This is augmented by an in-depth look at the role of sarcopenia, and frailty, which is reviewed in an excellent article by Drs Lucero and Verna, looking at the impact of protein restriction, malnourishment, and its resultant muscle wasting on HE and its management. Ammonia has been long recognized as a marker for encephalopathy; however, the difficulties in interpreting ammonia levels have cast questions on its absolute role. The difficulties in measuring ammonia, the role of measuring ammonia, and its role in pathogenesis are reviewed by Drs Parekh and Balart, and novel agents that are currently approved or in testing to lower ammonia are discussed by Drs Rahimi and Rockey. The cornerstones of treatment of our most significant clinical problems, overt encephalopathy and the encephalopathy in acute hepatic failure, are discussed in excellent articles by Dr Sussman and Drs Kodali and McGuire, respectively.

Clin Liver Dis 19 (2015) xi–xii
http://dx.doi.org/10.1016/j.cld.2015.05.004
1089-3261/15/$ – see front matter © 2015 Published by Elsevier Inc.

Finally, the vexing questions about legal and ethical responsibilities for patients with HE, in particular, their ability to drive, are discussed in Dr Vierling's fascinating review of the legal implications, including the state regulations on reporting of HE, both for ability to operate a motor vehicle and for other legal responsibilities. Overall, this issue of *Clinics in Liver Disease* takes an old problem and views it in a new light with the new diagnostic approaches, new understanding of pathogenesis, as well as new and emerging therapeutics, which I am certain will enhance our readers' clinical knowledge and their management of this challenging clinical problem.

Many people need to be acknowledged in the production of this issue. First, I am thankful to my authors, who have produced what I think is top-flight material throughout, giving new views to every topic. I would like to thank the publisher, and in particular, Meredith Clinton, without whose ongoing support and holding me to task on timelines, this probably never would have been done. I am sorry for all the times that I was late. Last, and most importantly, I would like to thank my family: my children, Bella, Jake, Dylan, Jacqueline, and Peyton, and my lovely wife, Sarah. Though my love for you makes it hard to leave each day to go to work, it also inspires me to try to do great things.

Robert S. Brown Jr, MD, MPH
Division of Gastroenterology and Hepatology
Weill Cornell Medical College
Center for Liver Disease and Transplantation
1305 York Avenue, 4th Floor
New York, NY 10021, USA

E-mail address:
rsb2005@med.cornell.edu

New Methods of Testing and Brain Imaging in Hepatic Encephalopathy: A Review

Raja G.R. Edula, MD, MRCP (UK),
Nikolaos T. Pyrsopoulos, MD, PhD, MBA*

KEYWORDS

- Hepatic encephalopathy • Ammonia • Psychometric testing • Stroop app
- Brain imaging • Magnetic resonance spectroscopy • Single-photon emission CT
- PET

KEY POINTS

- Hepatic encephalopathy (HE) is a clinical diagnosis requiring the exclusion of other causes of altered cerebral function.
- Diagnosis requires the presence of decompensated cirrhosis, acute liver failure, acute-on-chronic liver failure, or portosystemic shunting without cirrhosis.
- Psychometric tests are useful in the diagnosis of covert HE (CHE) but can be expensive and time consuming.
- Serum ammonia measurement is not routinely recommended for diagnosis.
- Functional brain imaging plays an important role in the diagnosis and understanding the pathogenesis of HE.

INTRODUCTION

HE comprises a spectrum of neuropsychiatric manifestations that can occur in patients with cirrhosis, acute liver failure, acute-on-chronic liver failure, or major portosystemic shunting without intrinsic liver disease.[1] It is characterized by disturbances in cognitive and motor function that can manifest as a change in personality, altered mood, diminished intellectual capacity, abnormal muscle tone, and tremor, among other symptoms in chronic liver disease.[2] The manifestations of this entity in acute liver failure can include abrupt-onset delirium, seizures, and coma as a result of cerebral

The Authors have nothing to disclose.
Division of Gastroenterology & Hepatology, Rutgers New Jersey Medical School, 185 South Orange Avenue, MSB H 538, Newark, NJ 07103, USA
* Corresponding author. Rutgers New Jersey Medical School, Medical Science Building (MSB), 185 South Orange Avenue, Room H- 538, Newark, NJ 07101.
E-mail address: pyrsopni@njms.rutgers.edu

Clin Liver Dis 19 (2015) 449–459
http://dx.doi.org/10.1016/j.cld.2015.04.001
1089-3261/15/$ – see front matter © 2015 Elsevier Inc. All rights reserved.

edema, increased intracranial pressure, and eventually brain herniation as a terminal event.[3,4] Early symptoms of HE might be subtle in nature and require psychometric testing to be identified.[5] Clinically obvious psychomotor derangements may occur later on as the disease progresses. Hence, it is imperative to identify these subtle manifestations to facilitate early diagnosis.[5] A diagnosis of HE is mainly clinical and usually made by the exclusion of other causes of brain or spinal cord dysfunction and proved by response to available therapy.[5] Certain imaging characteristics, such as basal ganglia hyperintensity on T1-weighted MRIs, are present in patients with end-stage liver disease, pointing toward the diagnosis, but are not pathognomic for HE.[6] Functional brain imaging is valuable and has provided important information into the understanding of the pathophysiology of HE but an optimal, clinically relevant and easily accessible test remains elusive.[7]

DIAGNOSING HEPATIC ENCEPHALOPATHY

To suspect a diagnosis of HE, as the term implies, a clinician has to first identify the presence of cirrhosis, acute liver failure, or portosystemic shunts without intrinsic liver disease. Testing should include methods for diagnosing CHE and overt HE.[5] Early symptoms include cognitive deficits in attention, visual perception, visuospatial construction, motor speed, and accuracy.[8] The subtle nature of these deficits can require psychometric testing for diagnosis. Clinically obvious symptoms and signs occur later on as the disease is advancing but a diagnosis can be made only after exclusion of other causes of cerebral dysfunction.[5] Additional diagnostic approaches include biochemical analysis to determine serum ammonia levels, brain imaging, electroencephalogram (EEG), lumbar puncture (LP), and other new methods of functional brain imaging, like magnetic resonance spectroscopy (MRS), PET, and single-photon emission computed tomography (SPECT).[5]

PSYCHOMETRIC TESTS

Hamster and colleagues[9] paved the way for further standardization in testing methods for CHE; 96 cirrhotic patients and 163 healthy age-matched controls were subjected to more than 30 different psychometric tests to assess cognitive domains ranging from premorbid intelligence levels to verbal abilities to visuomotor function and to coordination. It was published that the line tracing test, pegboard, aiming and steadiness of motor performance scale, and digit symbol test could effectively differentiate cirrhotic and noncirrhotic patients. CHE patients show abnormalities, particularly in areas of attention (loss of vigilance and disorientation), executive functions (problem solving, planning, and judgment), visuospatial coordination, and psychomotor speed (reaction times).[10] Underlying many of these deficits is an impaired response inhibition.[11] Psychometric testing strategies focus on defining abnormalities related to these domains using neuropsychological or neurophysiologic tests.[11] An overall brief description of available psychometric tests and their practical application in diagnosis of CHE are depicted in **Table 1**.

The drawbacks of applying psychometric tests in CHE patients include time and effort added to outpatient visits, lack of standardization, reliance on psychological expertise to administer and interpret results, the expensive and copyrighted testing procedures involved in the application of these tests, and potential reimbursement issues.[12]

STROOP APPLICATION

The Stroop smartphone application (app), which was developed by Bajaj and colleagues,[13] is a short and recently validated test to screen and diagnose patients

Table 1
Available psychometric tests

Test	Domain Tested	Comments
Paper-and-pencil psychometric tests		
Number connection test, part A	Psychomotor speed	Poor specificity
Number connection test, part B	Psychomotor speed	More specific
Digital symbol test	Psychomotor speed/attention	Very sensitive
Serial dotting test	Psychomotor speed	Psychomotor speed only
Block design test	Psychomotor speed	Lasts 20 min
Line tracing test	Psychomotor speed	Speed and accuracy
Repeatable battery for the assessment of neuropsychological status	Psychomotor speed	Used in dementia and brain injury
Computerized psychometric tests		
Inhibitory control test	Attention, vigilance, working memory	Requires highly functional patient, computer skilled
Cognitive drug research	Attention + episodic + working memory	Requires highly functional patient, computer skilled
Stern paradigm	Working memory, vigilance, attention	—
Neuropsychological tests		
EEG mean dominant frequency	Generalized brain activity	Can be performed in comatose patients
Visual evoked potentials	Interval between visual stimulus and activity	Highly variable, poor results
Brainstem auditory evoked potentials	Response in the cortex after auditory click stimuli	Inconsistent response
Critical flicker frequency	Visual discrimination and general arousal	Requires highly functional patients

Adapted from Montgomery JY, Bajaj JS. Diagnosis of minimal hepatic encephalopathy. In: Mullen KD, Prakash RK, editors. Hepatic Encephalopathy. Berlin: Humana Press/Springer; 2012. p. 103–12.

with CHE. It is marketed as the EncephalApp—Stroop Test (available as a free download on iTunes). The app is easy to administer and quick to teach patients, and the interpretation is simple without the need for a psychologist to administer the test. EncephalApp has an on state, which is a measure of response inhibition and motor speed, and an off state, which assesses psychomotor ability. The results measured include off time (total time required to complete 5 correct runs in the off state), on time (total time required to complete 5 correct runs in the on state), off time plus on time, and the number of runs required to complete 5 correct off and on runs by the subject. Both components were administered to subjects after 2 training runs were given for each state.

During validation of the test, all patients with cirrhosis performed worse on standard paper-and-pencil psychometric tests and EncephalApp tests compared with controls. Patients with cirrhosis and overt HE performed worse than those without overt HE. An off time plus on time value of greater than 190 seconds identified all patients with CHE.

EncephalApp times also correlated with accidents and illegal turns in driving simulation tests. It was determined that the app has good face validity, test-retest reliability, and external validity for diagnosis of CHE. Use of this app may facilitate the evaluation and treatment of patients with CHE in the United States, where testing for this stage of HE is not routinely administered.

AMMONIA

Measurement of serum ammonia levels may be helpful in the initial evaluation of patients with altered mental status, when the presence of significant liver disease has not been established and other causes are suspected.[14] The diagnostic value of ammonia is limited by several factors. Levels can be influenced by potential errors associated with sample collection, handling, and storage.[15] Artifactual increase in ammonia levels can be seen in patients with mild exertion prior to sampling and spontaneous release of ammonia from red blood cells in blood samples left at room temperature.[16] In patients with acute liver failure, elevated levels of arterial ammonia (>150 mg/dL) have been associated with an increased risk of complications and cerebral herniation.[17,18] In patients with cirrhosis, no consistent correlation between serum ammonia level, risk of cerebral edema, and severity of HE has been identified.[19]

Blood for ammonia level should be collected from a stasis-free vein. Avoid fist clenching or application of a tourniquet, which can elevate ammonia levels due to release from skeletal muscle. Blood should be collected in a lithium heparin– or sodium heparin–containing (green top) Vacutainer because heparin inhibits the release of ammonia from red blood cells. Samples should be stored and transported in an ice bath and tested within 20 minutes for ammonia assay.[20]

Measurement of serum ammonia levels alone might not be a definitive diagnostic tool for HE and is not indicated for routine diagnosis in daily clinical practice.[5] Other metabolic disturbances that may affect the cerebral function, including hyponatremia[21] in cirrhotic patients and hypoglycemia in patients with acute liver failure,[22] need to be considered.

BRAIN IMAGING

Clinicians working with patients suffering from HE currently have to accept that there are no specific imaging or clinical findings that ensure the diagnosis. If a patient with liver disease presents with neuropsychiatric aberrations, a diagnosis of HE has to be considered after excluding other possible causes. Therefore, in clinical practice, CT and MRI of the brain are used to exclude other causes of cerebral dysfunction, including intracranial hemorrhage, infarction, infection, or tumor. Although CT scan findings are usually unremarkable, subtle abnormalities have been observed in cirrhotic patients without HE that suggest frontal cortical atrophy and mild cerebral edema.[23] Conventional T1 or T2 MRI is available in most centers and allows exclusion of other neurologic diseases and may reveal typical signs of HE.[24] A majority of patients with cirrhosis or portosystemic shunts exhibit bilateral, symmetric high signal intensity at the globus pallidus and substantia nigra.[25] This signal may increase after transjugular intrahepatic portosystemic shunt placement[26] and reverses after occlusion of congenital portosystemic shunts.[27] Rise in concentration of manganese, a paramagnetic substance in the central nervous system, with preferential deposition in the globus pallidus, is the most possible explanation for this finding.[28,29] Although pallidal hyperintensities are found in 90% of cirrhotic patients, they are not closely linked to the presence of HE.[30] It has been demonstrated that cirrhotic patients with no clinical or neuropsychiatric signs of HE can also show severe signal alterations, whereas others with HE may present with slight signal alterations only.[30–32] Clinical experience, however, indicates that the absence of T1 high signal intensity on MRI is a strong indicator against interpreting neurologic manifestations as secondary to liver disease.[10]

LUMBAR PUNCTURE

Unlike brain imaging, fluid analysis of cerebrospinal fluid obtained from LP is not required for diagnosis of HE but may be necessary when other conditions, such as meningitis, encephalitis, and subarachnoid hemorrhage, are suspected. Moreover, patients with liver disease may present with severe coagulopathy and decreased platelet count, and LP is often contraindicated due to risk of bleeding. In addition patients with acute liver failure might suffer from cerebral edema and increased intracranial pressure and are at a risk of brainstem herniation subsequent to the procedure. When performed to exclude other comorbidities in patients with HE, however, increased levels of cerebrospinal fluid glutamine concentrations as well as an increase in aromatic amino acids have been identified.[33]

ELECTROENCEPHALOGRAM

EEG provides useful information to quantify brain dysfunction in HE. More than 50 years ago, Parsons-Smith and colleagues[34] showed that EEG patterns have an approximate relationship with behavioral features of HE. The first EEG sign of HE is a low-frequency alpha rhythm disturbed by random waves in the theta region over both cerebral hemispheres.[35] Increases in the severity of HE induce progressive increases in the theta band activity along with high-voltage delta band activity. Triphasic waves can be seen at this stage although they are not specific to HE and can be observed in other types of metabolic encephalopathy.[36–38] In comatose patients, the tracings are formed by high-voltage arrhythmic delta waves and finally a flat EEG.[39] Once a flat EEG is reached, further information of brain activity can be obtained by somatosensory evoked potentials.[40] EEG quantification provides good assessment of risk for developing overt HE and mortality at 1-year follow-up in patients who do not display symptoms of overt encephalopathy at the time of examination.[41] EEG, thus, is a valuable tool in clinical practice to investigate HE. Although to a lesser extent than clinical grading of HE, inter- and intraobserver variability does exist with EEG. With cartography of cerebral electrical activity, or brain mapping, EEG can analyze various regions of the brain. This technique has high sensitivity for functional alterations of the brain, and 85% of patients with no clinical symptoms of HE show abnormalities on this technique.[42] This technology also serves to simplify the interpretation of EEG.

The interpretation of EEG findings is independent of patient's cooperation and education level. On the contrary, psychometric testing is influenced by patient education and cooperation. EEG might be considered a complementary test. In CHE, it has proved to have a higher predictive value on survival compared with psychometric testing.[43] EEG can objectively depict changes in brain function after treatment and can be a useful follow-up test to assess treatment response.[44] It has been reported that there is prognostic value of the EEG findings for the development of HE and mortality in cirrhotic patients.[45] Marked improvement in EEG findings has also been demonstrated in the post-transplant setting[46] and may play a role in the evaluation of post-transplant neurologic complications.[47]

MAGNETIC RESONANCE SPECTROSCOPY

MRS has been widely used in recent times for the evaluation of HE as a result of improved sequence development and higher field strength to resolve metabolite signals. The technique is based on the same physical principles as MRI and the detection of energy exchange between external magnetic fields and specific nuclei within atoms. MRS can be performed with existing MRI equipment and modified with additional software and hardware. It is considered investigational and not routinely available for clinical use.

MRS facilitates the investigation of HE and effects of increased ammonia supply and metabolism in the cerebral tissue in vivo at the molecular level.[6] MRS detects the relaxation properties of some atoms in strong magnetic fields and can generate high-resolution images or spectrum of several metabolites that contain the atoms studied.[48] A series of metabolites is displayed as peaks at different frequencies in the spectrum. Hydrogen proton-MRS demonstrates relative to creatinine an increase in glutamine/glutamate (Glx) signal and a decrease of choline (cho)-containing compounds and myo-inositol.[49] Abnormalities in the Glx signal have been interpreted as an increase in brain glutamine secondary to metabolism of ammonia in the astrocyte. Disturbances of cho and myo-inositol have been interpreted as a compensatory response to increase in intracellular osmolality caused by accumulation of glutamine in astrocytes.[48]

The severity of changes seen in MRS have been proposed as a signature of HE based on studies.[50] In patients with cirrhosis subjected to ammonia load, hydrogen proton-MRS consistently showed increase in Glx signal accompanied by myo-inositol depletion and decrease in the cho signal in all regions.[51–53] These changes are considered to reflect basic metabolic alterations of the brain in cirrhotics that are involved in the development of HE.[54] In a study performed in patients with minimal HE, a decrease in myo-inositol was the most accurate predictor of minimal HE compared with MRI or psychometric tests.[55] The evolution of hydrogen proton-MRS abnormalities after liver transplantation and their reversibility have been assessed in longitudinal studies.[30,31] This reversibility precedes the disappearance of pallidal hyperintensity after liver transplantation and correlates with clinical neurologic improvement.[56]

The extent of MRS changes increase with increasing grade of encephalopathy.[57] These changes have also been observed in cirrhotic patients, with neither clinical nor psychomotor signs of cerebral dysfunction.[48] Patients with Child class C cirrhosis with and without HE did not differ with regard to findings on MRS.[58] The characteristic MRS changes seem to reflect metabolic alterations more than functional alterations of the brain and are not perfect indicators of HE. Therefore, MRS alterations cannot be used as a sole test to diagnose HE.

SINGLE-PHOTON EMISSION COMPUTED TOMOGRAPHY

SPECT studies the spatial distribution of radioactive tracer technetium Tc 99 and its local metabolism in the brain. Because these radionuclides are uncommon to human body, the tracer binding or metabolization may not be identical to that of native molecule and, hence, difficulties in the interpretation of results can occur.[59] Previous studies have shown increased blood flow in the basal ganglia of patients with minimal HE, suggesting increased ammonia delivery to these areas, resulting in astrocyte dysfunction and cognitive impairment.[60,61] SPECT provides only relative measurements of radioactivity and allows the comparison of physiologic parameters like blood flow in different areas of the brain.

Compared with PET, discussed later, this method is more easily available and less expensive. PET is preferred in functional imaging studies of the brain, however, due to its superior spatial resolution.[62] Studies that have investigated SPECT in HE have been limited by small study sizes, limiting the use of this tool in diagnosis of HE.

PET

PET is a nuclear imaging test based on the detection of positron emission associated with isotope decay. The 4 main isotopes used for clinical purposes are oxygen

15 (^{15}O), nitrogen 13 (^{13}N), carbon 11 (^{11}C), and fluorine 18 (^{18}F).[63] Using these isotopes, a large number of tracers can be synthesized to study brain function. In patients with cirrhosis and HE, the tracers used ^{15}O-H_2O, ^{13}N-amonia (NH_3), and ^{18}F-fluorodeoxyglu-cose (FDG). PET has the ability to obtain quantitative data of isotope distribution and use the data with measurements of radioactivity in the blood to calculate physiologic parameters like blood flow, glucose metabolism, and ammonia metabolism.[57] PET has been applied to investigate the cerebral ammonia metabolism in parallel with cere-bral glucose utilization.[64] In this study, plasma ammonia levels correlated with ammonia metabolism of the brain and with MRS in white matter. MRS also showed a correlation with cerebral glucose utilization. Ammonia metabolism and glucose utilization were, however, not associated. The study suggests that cerebral ammonia metabolism is important in the development of HE but is not the only factor.

Oxygen consumption and cerebral blood flow have been investigated in cirrhotic pa-tients with and without HE and compared with healthy controls.[65] A decrease in oxygen consumption and cerebral blood flow was induced by HE. It has been proposed that the inability to use delivered oxygen of patients with HE relates to a specific inhibition asso-ciated with oxidative metabolism in mitochondria.[66] Lockwood and colleagues[67] have used FDG-PET to investigate functional changes in HE. They were able to demonstrate a reduction in glucose metabolism in the anterior cingulate gyrus, which may reflect attention deficit found in HE patients on neuropsychiatric testing and in functional mag-netic resonance studies. Alteration in cerebral blood flow has also been established us-ing FDG-PET and ^{15}O-PET, where poor neuropsychiatric test performance correlated with reduced blood flow in all cortical areas. Temporal lobe blood flow was found most discriminatory between HE patients and healthy volunteers.[68]

A disadvantage of PET is its limited spatial resolution and the lack of information about the anatomic structures represented by the detected metabolic data. These dis-advantages can be overcome by coregistration of PET images and MRIs of a patient and defining regions of interest, based on anatomic information provided by MRI before further analysis of the PET data.[57] Possible clinical implications of PET is in the differential diagnosis with other neurologic disorders, like Alzheimer or Parkinson disease, for which specific radioligands are available.[69]

PET and SPECT have provided valuable insight into the pathogenesis of HE but are not widely available diagnostic tools. Their use in the evaluation of HE is limited by the expense and availability of the tests and currently limited to research based academic centers. Promising functional data are emerging, but standardization in regard to uni-formity of study protocols, imaging sequences, and analysis methods is required before they become widely available diagnostic tools for HE,[7] which is a common but under-recognized complication of cirrhosis.

SUMMARY

Despite several advances in diagnostic testing of HE, it remains a clinical diagnosis based on clinical criteria that classify HE into various grades ranging from normal mental status to coma. Because this clinical classification is somewhat subjective, additional diagnostic tools are required. Subtle memory and attention deficits in cir-rhotics are not always caused by HE and adequate diagnostic tests are required. Although ammonia levels are routinely measured in patients with altered conscious-ness, elevated levels do not always result in HE even in the presence of cirrhosis. Further testing is required to clarify the diagnosis and exclude other causes. Psycho-metric tests are used to diagnose minimal HE, although correction may be required for age and educational level and they are not routinely used in clinical practice. The

Stroop smartphone app is a short and validated psychometric test that recently has become available to assist in identifying patients with CHE. Brain imaging is used mainly to rule out other causes; although some MRI findings are characteristic in patients with cirrhosis, they are not pathognomic of HE.

New neuroimaging techniques, especially functional brain imaging, have seen rapid development in recent years, and the data obtained from the brains of patients with different stages of liver disease have provided a better understanding of the pathogenesis. It is now known that the pattern of cerebral dysfunction in HE is restricted to certain brain anatomic structures and functional circuits involving specific metabolites, at least in the early stages of the disease. Although these tests are not standardized in terms of applying them to routine clinical practice, extensive information obtained from the use of these modalities supports their use in monitoring and evaluating the effect of current and new therapeutic agents for HE, and they may become standard of care in the near future.

REFERENCES

1. Ferenci P, Lockwood A, Mullen K, et al. Hepatic encephalopathy definition, nomenclature, diagnosis and quantification: final report of the working party at the 11th world congress of Gastroenterology, Vienna, 1998. Hepatology 2002;35(3):716–21.
2. Lockwood AH. Hepatic encephalopathy. Boston: Butterworth-Heinemann; 1992.
3. Ede RJ, Williams R. Hepatic encephalopathy and cerebral edema. Semin Liver Dis 1986;6:107–18.
4. Hoofnagle JH, Carithers RL Jr, Shapiro C, et al. Fulminant hepatic failure: summary of a workshop. Hepatology 1995;21:240–52.
5. Weissenborn K. Diagnosis of overt hepatic encephalopathy. In: Mullen KD, Prakash RK, editors. Hepatic Encephalopathy. Berlin: Humana Press/Springer; 2012. p. 97–102.
6. McPhail MJ, Taylor-Robinson S. The role of magnetic resonance imaging and spectroscopy in hepatic encephalopathy. Metab Brain Dis 2010;25(1):65–72.
7. Mcphail MJ, Patel NR, Taylor-Robinson SD. Brain imaging and hepatic encephalopathy. Clin Liver Dis 2012;1:57–72.
8. Weissenborn K, Ennen JC, Schomerus H, et al. Neuropsychological characterization of hepatic encephalopathy. J Hepatol 2001;34:768–73.
9. Schomerus H, Hamster W. Neuropsychological aspects of porto-systemic encephalopathy. Metab Brain Dis 1998;13(4):361–77.
10. Cordoba J. New assessment of hepatic encephalopathy. J Hepatol 2011;54(5):1030–40.
11. Bajaj JS, Wade JB, Sanyal AJ. Spectrum of neurocognitive impairment in cirrhosis: implications for the assessment of hepatic encephalopathy. Hepatology 2009;50(6):2014–21.
12. Bajaj JS, Etemadian A, Hafeezullah M, et al. Testing for minimal hepatic encephalopathy in the United States: an AASLD survey. Hepatology 2007;45(3):833–4.
13. Bajaj JS, Thacker LR, Heuman DM, et al. The stroop smartphone application is a short and valid method to screen for minimal hepatic encephalopathy. Hepatology 2013;58(3):1122–32.
14. Mullen KD, Ferenci F, Bass N, et al. An algorithm for the management of hepatic encephalopathy. Semin Liver Dis 2007;27(2):32–47.
15. Howanitz JH, Howanitz PJ, Skrodzki CA, et al. Influences of specimen processing and storage conditions on results for plasma ammonia. Clin Chem 1984;30:906–8.

16. Barsotti RJ. Measurement of ammonia in blood. J Pediatr 2001;138:S11–9.
17. Bhatia V, Singh R, Acharya SK. Predictive value of arterial ammonia for complications and outcome in acute liver failure. Gut 2006;55:98–104.
18. Clemmesen JO, Larsen FS, Kondrup J, et al. Cerebral herniation in patients with acute liver failure is correlated with arterial ammonia concentration. Hepatology 1999;29:648–53.
19. Kundra A, Jain A, Banga A, et al. Evaluation of plasma ammonia levels in patients with acute liver failure and chronic liver disease and its correlation with the severity of hepatic encephalopathy and clinical features of raised intracranial tension. Clin Biochem 2005;38:696–9.
20. Prakash RK, Mullen K. Hepatic encephalopathy. Schiff's Diseases of the Liver, vol. 18. Chichester, UK: Wiley-Blackwell; 2012. p. 421–43.
21. Córdoba J, García-Martinez R, Simón-Talero M. Hyponatremia and hepatic encephalopathies: similarities, differences and coexistence. Metab Brain Dis 2010;25(1):75–80.
22. Bernal W, Auzinger G, Dhawan A, et al. Acute liver failure. Lancet 2010;376: 190–201.
23. Bernthal P, Hays A, Tarter RE, et al. Cerebral CT scan abnormalities in cholestatic and hepatocellular disease and their relationship to neuropsychological test performance. Hepatology 1987;7:107–14.
24. Cordoba J, Minguez B. Hepatic encephalopathy. Semin Liver Dis 2008;28(1): 70–80.
25. Pujol A, Pujol J, Graus F, et al. Hyperintense globus pallidus on T1-weighted MRI in cirrhotic patients is associated with severity of liver failure. Neurology 1993; 43(1):65–9.
26. Matsumoto S, Mori H, Yoshioka K, et al. Effects of portal-systemic shunt embolization on the basal ganglia: MRI. Neuroradiology 1997;39(5):326–8.
27. Butterworth RF, Spahr L, Fontaine S, et al. Manganese toxicity, dopaminergic dysfunction and hepatic encephalopathy. Metab Brain Dis 1995;10(4):259–67.
28. Spahr L, Butterworth RF, Fontaine S, et al. Increased blood manganese in cirrhotic patients: relationship to pallidal magnetic resonance signal hyperintensity and neurological symptoms. Hepatology 1996;24(5):1116–20.
29. Pomier-Layrargues G, Spahr L, Butterworth RF. Increased manganese concentrations in pallidum of cirrhotic patients. Lancet 1995;345(8951):735.
30. Cordoba J, Olive G, Alonso J, et al. Improvement of magnetic resonance spectroscopic abnormalities but not pallidal hyperintensity followed amelioration of hepatic encephalopathy after occlusion of a large spleno-renal shunt. J Hepatol 2001;34(1):176–8.
31. Cordoba J, Alonso J, Rovira A, et al. The development of low-grade cerebral edema in cirrhosis is supported by the evolution of (1) H-magnetic resonance abnormalities after liver transplantation. J Hepatol 2001;35(5):598–604.
32. Naegele T, Grodd W, Viebahn R, et al. MR imaging and (1)Hspectroscopy of brain metabolites in hepatic encephalopathy: time-course of renormalization after liver transplantation. Radiology 2000;216(3):683–91.
33. Hourani B, Hamlin E, Reynolds T. Cerebrospinal fluid glutamine as a measure of hepatic encephalopathy. Arch Intern Med 1971;172:1033–6.
34. Parsons-Smith BG, Summerskill WH, Dawson AM, et al. The electroencephalograph in liver disease. Lancet 1957;2:867–71.
35. Montagnese S, Jackson C, Morgan MY. Spatio-temporal decomposition of the electroencephalogram in patients with cirrhosis. J Hepatol 2007;46(3): 447–58.

36. Bickford RG, Butt HR. Hepatic coma: the electroencephalographic pattern. J Clin Invest 1955;34:790–6.
37. Kaplan PW. The EEG in metabolic encephalopathy and coma. J Clin Neurophysiol 2004;21(5):307–18.
38. Karnaze DS, Bickford RG. Triphasic waves: a reassessment of their significance. Electroencephalogr Clin Neurophysiol 1984;57(3):193–8.
39. Amodio P, Gatta A. Neurophysiological investigation of hepatic encephalopathy. Metab Brain Dis 2005;20(4):369–79.
40. Guerit JM, Amantini A, Fischer C, et al. Neurophysiological investigations of hepatic encephalopathy: ISHEN practice guidelines. Liver Int 2009;29(6):789–96.
41. Amodio P, Marchetti P, Del Piccolo F, et al. Spectral versus visual EEG analysis in mild hepatic encephalopathy. Clin Neurophysiol 1999;110(8):1334–44.
42. Kullmann F, Hollerbach S, Lock G, et al. Brain electrical activity mapping of EEG for the diagnosis of (sub)clinical hepatic encephalopathy in chronic liver disease. Eur J Gastroenterol Hepatol 2001;13:513–22.
43. Saxena N, Bhatia M, Joshi YK, et al. Electrophysiological and neuropsychological tests for the diagnosis of subclinical hepatic encephalopathy and prediction of overt encephalopathy. Liver 2002;22(3):190–7.
44. Amodio P. The electroencephalogram in hepatic encephalopathy. In: Mullen KD, Prakash RK, editors. Hepatic Encephalopathy. Berlin: Humana Press/Springer; 2012. p. 113–21.
45. Amodio P, Del Piccolo F, Petteno E, et al. Prevalence and prognostic value of quantified electroencephalogram (EEG) alterations in cirrhotic patients. J Hepatol 2001;35:37–45.
46. Epstein CM, Riether AM, Henderson RM, et al. EEG in liver transplantation: visual and computerized analysis. Electroencephalogr Clin Neurophysiol 1992;83(6):367–71.
47. Steg RE, Wszolek ZK. Electroencephalographic abnormalities in liver transplant recipients: practical considerations and review. J Clin Neurophysiol 1996;13(1):60–8.
48. Garcia-Martinez R, Cordoba J. Brain imaging in hepatic encephalopathy. In: Mullen KD, Prakash RK, editors. Hepatic Encephalopathy. Berlin: Humana Press/Springer; 2012. p. 123–37.
49. Kostler H. Proton magnetic resonance spectroscopy in portal-systemic encephalopathy. Metab Brain Dis 1998;13(4):291–301.
50. Geissler A, Lock G, Frund R, et al. Cerebral abnormalities in patients with cirrhosis detected by proton magnetic resonance spectroscopy and magnetic resonance imaging. Hepatology 1997;25(1):48–54.
51. Kreis R, Ross BD, Farrow NA, et al. Metabolic disorders of the brain in chronic hepatic encephalopathy detected with H-1 MR spectroscopy. Radiology 1992;182(1):19–27.
52. Cordoba J. Glutamine, myo-inositol, and brain edema in acute liver failure. Hepatology 1996;23(5):1291–2.
53. Thomas MA, Huda A, Guze B, et al. Cerebral 1H MR spectroscopy and neuropsychologic status of patients with hepatic encephalopathy. AJR Am J Roentgenol 1998;171(4):1123–30.
54. Haussinger D, Laubenberger J, Vom Dahl S, et al. Proton magnetic resonance spectroscopy studies on human brain myo-inositol in hypo-osmolarity and hepatic encephalopathy. Gastroenterology 1994;107(5):1475–80.
55. Singhal A, Nagarajan R, Hinkin CH, et al. Two dimensional MR spectroscopy of minimal hepatic encephalopathy and neuropsychological correlates in vivo. J Magn Reson Imaging 2010;32(1):35–43.

56. Cordoba J, Raguer N, Flavia M, et al. T2 hyperintensity along the cortico-spinal tract in cirrhosis relates to functional abnormalities. Hepatology 2003;38(4): 1026–33.

57. Weissenborn K, Bokemeyer M, Ahl B, et al. Functional imaging of the brain in patients with liver cirrhosis. Metab Brain Dis 2004;19:269–80.

58. Lee JH, Seo DW, Lee YS, et al. Proton magnetic resonance spectroscopy findings in the brain in patients with liver cirrhosis reflect the hepatic functional reserve. Am J Gastroenterol 1999;94(8):2206–13.

59. Lammertsma AA. PET/SPECT: functional imaging beyond flow. Vis Res 2001;41: 1277–81.

60. O'Carroll RE. Regional cerebral blood flow and cognitive function in patients with chronic liver disease. Lancet 1991;337(8752):1250.

61. Catafau AM. Relationship between cerebral perfusion in frontal-limbic-basal ganglia circuits and neuropsychologic impairment in patients with subclinical hepatic encephalopathy. J Nucl Med 2000;41(3):405.

62. Stewart C, Reivich M, Lucey M, et al. Neuroimaging in hepatic encephalopathy. Clin Gastroenterol Hepatol 2005;3(3):197–207.

63. Miller PW. Synthesis of 11C, 18F, 15O, and 13N radiolabels for positron emission tomography. Angew Chem Int Ed Engl 2008;47(47):8998.

64. Weissenborn K, Ahl B, Fischer-Wasels D, et al. Correlations between magnetic resonance spectroscopy alterations and cerebral ammonia and glucose metabolism in cirrhotic patients with and without hepatic encephalopathy. Gut 2007; 56(12):1736–42.

65. Iversen P, Sorensen M, Bak LK, et al. Low cerebral oxygen consumption and blood flow in patients with cirrhosis and an acute episode of hepatic encephalopathy. Gastroenterology 2009;136(3):863–71.

66. Keiding S, Sorensen M, Munk OL, et al. Human (13)N-ammonia PET studies: the importance of measuring (13)N-ammonia metabolites in blood. Metab Brain Dis 2010;25(1):49–56.

67. Lockwood AH, Weissenborn K, Bokemeyer M, et al. Correlations between cerebral glucose metabolism and neuropsychological test performance in nonalcoholic cirrhotics. Metab Brain Dis 2002;17(1):29–40.

68. Lockwood AH. Altered cerebral blood flow and glucose metabolism in patients with liver disease and minimal encephalopathy. J Cereb Blood Flow Metab 1991;11(2):331.

69. Narendran R, Mason NS, Laymon CM, et al. A comparative evaluation of the dopamine D (2/3) agonist radiotracer [11C] (-)-N-propylnorapomorphine and antagonist [11C] raclopride to measure amphetamine-induced dopamine release in the human striatum. J Pharmacol Exp Ther 2010;333(2):533–9.

Clinical and Neurologic Manifestation of Minimal Hepatic Encephalopathy and Overt Hepatic Encephalopathy

 CrossMark

P. Patrick Basu, MD, MRCP[a,b], Niraj James Shah, MD[c],*

KEYWORDS

- Neurologic manifestation • Minimal hepatic encephalopathy • MHE
- Overt hepatic encephalopathy • OHE

KEY POINTS

- Hepatic encephalopathy shows a wide spectrum of neuropsychiatric manifestations, whereas minimal hepatic encephalopathy (MHE) is largely under-recognized.
- Subtle symptoms of MHE can only be diagnosed through specialized neuropsychiatric testing.
- Early diagnosis and treatment may drastically improve the quality of life for many cirrhotic patients.

INTRODUCTION

Hepatic encephalopathy (HE) shows a wide spectrum of neuropsychiatric manifestations.[1] With progression, personality changes occur, such as apathy, irritability, and disinhibition, along with obvious alternations in mental status and motor functions.[2] During the course of the disorder, patients develop altered mental status with disorientation, inappropriate behavior, memory impairment, shortened attention span, slurred speech, confusion and eventually coma.[3] Sleep disturbances with changes in the sleep-wake cycle and daytime somnolence occur early,[4] with later, less frequent

Disclosure: The authors have nothing to disclose.
[a] Department of Medicine, Columbia University College of Physicians and Surgeons, 622 West 168 Street, New York, NY 10032, USA; [b] Department of Medicine, King's County Hospital Medical Center, 450 Clarkson Avenue, Brooklyn, NY 11203, USA; [c] Department of Medicine, James J. Peters VA Medical Center, Icahn School of Medicine at Mount Sinai, 130 West Kingsbridge Road, New York, NY 10468, USA
* Corresponding author.
E-mail address: nirajjames@gmail.com

Clin Liver Dis 19 (2015) 461–472
http://dx.doi.org/10.1016/j.cld.2015.05.003
1089-3261/15/$ – see front matter © 2015 Elsevier Inc. All rights reserved.

liver.theclinics.com

reversal of the sleep-wake cycle.[5,6] Decompensated cirrhotics with portal hypertension have been reported to experience a higher incidence of restless legs syndrome.[7]

Patients, and often family members and friends, describe changes in memory, cognition, and behavior. Bizarre behavior and overt personality changes are more frequently reported than paranoia. Shortened attention span and mildly impaired

Table 1
HE: symptoms/grading

West-Haven Criteria (WHC) including MHE	ISHEN	Description	Suggested Operative Criteria	Comment
Unimpaired		No encephalopathy, no history of HE	Tested and proved to be normal	—
Minimal	Covert	Psychometric or neuropsychological alterations of tests exploring psychomotor speed/ executive functions or neurophysiologic alterations without clinical evidence of mental change	Abnormal results of established psychometric or neuropsychological tests without clinical manifestations	No universal criteria for diagnosis. Local standards and expertise required
Grade I		Trivial lack of awareness Euphoria or anxiety Shortened attention span Impairment of addition or subtraction Altered sleep rhythm	Despite oriented in time and space (discussed later), the patient seems to have some cognitive/behavioral decay with respect to the standard on clinical examination, or to the caregivers	Clinical findings usually not reproducible
Grade II	Overt	Lethargy or apathy Disorientation for time Obvious personality change Inappropriate behavior Dyspraxia Asterixis	Disoriented for time (at least 3 of the following are wrong: day of the month, day of the week, month, season, or year) ± the other mentioned symptoms	Clinical findings variable but reproducible to some extent
Grade III		Somnolence to semistupor Responsive to stimuli Confused Gross disorientation Bizarre behavior	Disoriented also for space (at least 3 of the following wrongly reported: country, state [or region], city or place) ± the other mentioned symptoms	Clinical findings reproducible to some extent
Grade IV		Coma	Does not respond even to pain stimuli	Comatose state usually reproducible

From American Association for the Study of Liver Diseases, European Association for the Study of the Liver. Hepatic encephalopathy in chronic liver disease: 2014 practice guideline by the European Association for the Study of the Liver and the American Association for the Study of Liver Diseases. J Hepatol 2014;61(3):645; with permission.

computations mark grade I HE. The patients themselves are often unaware of the subtle changes.

International Society for Hepatic Encephalopathy and Nitrogen Metabolism (ISHEN) consensus outlined the symptoms and their grading into covert (minimal HE [MHE] and grade I) and overt HE (OHE; grades II–IV) in September 2014[8] (**Table 1**). Impaired handwriting and incoordination initiate the motor manifestations of stage I HE. Asterixis signifies stage II HE. With progression of encephalopathy, the flapping tremors weaken in stage III before disappearing in stage IV. Hyporeflexia and ataxia later lead to hyperreflexia, clonus, and rigidity, ultimately resulting in opisthotonus and coma.

MHE is largely under-recognized. It negatively affects quality of life for patients and their families.[9] MHE is highly prevalent among patients with cirrhosis, affecting up to 80% of this population.[10] Patients with MHE have normal findings on clinical examination, but abnormal psychometric test results. Subtle symptoms of MHE can only be diagnosed through specialized neuropsychiatric testing.[1] This condition is best described as a disorder of executive functioning. Patients have deficits in vigilance, response inhibition, working memory, and orientation.[10] MHE has been shown to decrease quality of life and interfere with daily functioning, such as the ability to safely operate an automobile.[11] The recent ISHEN consensus uses the onset of disorientation or asterixis as the onset of OHE[12] (**Fig. 1**). As MHE is more widely recognized, its treatment may drastically improve the quality of life for many cirrhotic patients.

Recent understanding of the physiologic mechanisms for HE has helped clinicians to understand the signs and symptoms in various stages of HE. The blood-brain barrier (BBB) permeability of the cerebral cortex and cerebellum is different in different stages of HE. Although the BBB in the cerebellum is permeabilized from stage I of HE, the cerebrum's BBB is not affected (and hence has no vasogenic edema) until stage III of HE (**Fig. 2**).[13,14] The symptoms of HE are explained in **Table 2**.

Cirrhosis-associated parkinsonism, formerly known as acquired hepatolenticular degeneration, also occurs in chronic HE. Extrapyramidal symptoms are usually prominent compared with mental status changes and show partial overlap with

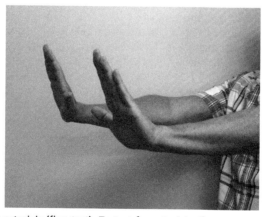

Fig. 1. Testing for asterixis (flap test). To test for asterixis, the arms are extended and the wrists dorsiflexed. (*Courtesy of* Hepatitis C Online/University of Washington. Available at: http://www.hepatitisc.uw.edu/go/management-cirrhosis-related-complications/hepatic-encephalopathy-diagnosis-management/core-concept/all. Accessed January 4, 2015.)

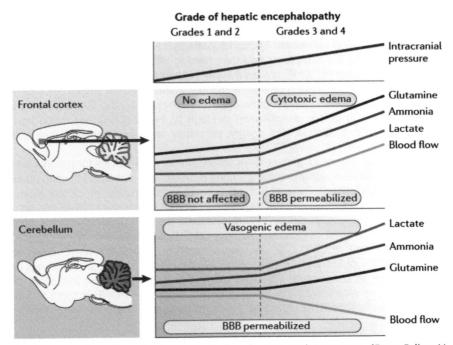

Fig. 2. Progression of cerebral and cerebellar changes and symptoms. (*From* Felipo V. Hepatic encephalopathy: effects of liver failure on brain function. Nat Rev Neurosci 2013;14(12):854; with permission.)

hepatic myelopathy.[32] It is usually unresponsive to ammonia level–lowering therapy and occurs in up to approximately 4% of patients with advanced liver disease.[33]

MECHANISM: MOTOR MANIFESTATIONS OF MINIMAL HEPATIC ENCEPHALOPATHY

Motor activation is induced by activation of the metabotropic glutamate receptors (mGluRs) in the nucleus accumbens (NAc)[14] (**Fig. 3**). The mechanism of this activation is different in rats with MHE (via glutamate) compared with control rats (via dopamine).[34] The neuroinflammation in MHE reduces the number and function of glutamate transporters[35]; reducing the activation of mGluRs in the NAc. This reduced activation leads to increased levels of extracellular gamma-aminobutyric acid (GABA), resulting in hypokinesia. Thus blocking glutamate receptors (stereotaxically with (E)-Ethyl 1,1a,7,7a-tetrahydro-7-(hydroxyimino)cyclopropa[b]chromene-1a-carboxylate (CPCCOEt), a noncompetitive antagonist at the glutamate receptor) restores motor activity.[36]

MECHANISM: COGNITIVE IMPAIRMENT IN MINIMAL HEPATIC ENCEPHALOPATHY

In rats with MHE, reduced synthesis of cyclase guanylyl monophosphate (cGMP) via various mechanisms results in impaired cognition, as shown by reduced learning ability in a Y maze task[14] (**Fig. 4**). Neuroinflammation (via increased extracellular GABA) and hyperammonemia (via increased activation of N-methyl-D-aspartate receptors); both ultimately reduce neuronal NO synthase, which results in reduced synthesis of cGMP.

Table 2
Symptoms explained

Symptom	Cause	Comments
Altered mental status, memory loss, disorientation, personality changes, memory impairment, shortened attention span, slurred speech, confusion, coma	Cerebral edema (varying degrees) with astrocyte swelling GABA toxic effects[15] Systemic inflammation[16] Alterations in the cerebral blood flux and in the oxidative metabolism[17]	Altered communication between the astrocyte and the neuron[18] Trojan horse theory: oxidative stress caused by mitochondrial ammonia accumulation (glutamate transport)[19]
Transient focal neurologic deficits or seizures	Cerebral edema (varying degrees) with astrocyte swelling GABA toxic effects[15] Alterations in the cerebral blood flux and in the oxidative metabolism[17]	Rarely occurs[20,21]
Asterixis (flapping tremors)	Abnormal function of diencephalic motor centers that regulate the tone of agonist and antagonist muscles, normally involved in maintaining posture[22]	Adams and Foley[23] first described asterixis in 1949 in patients with severe liver failure and encephalopathy Present in early to middle stages of HE Not pathognomonic; it occurs with renal failure, hypercapnia, and stroke affecting basal ganglia Asterixis does not occur in advanced HE Never seen in coma Testing for asterixis (see **Fig. 2**)
Hyperreflexia, hypertonia, or extensor plantar responses	Pyramidal involvement	Never seen in coma
Parkinsonian symptoms: bradykinesia, tremors	Deposition of manganese in the basal ganglia (globus pallidus and substantia nigra)[24]	Manganese induces changes in astrocytes of the basal ganglia that promote the formation of Alzheimer type II astrocytes Manganese acts as a neurotoxin to stimulate translocator proteins on astrocytes Tics or chorea are rare[25] Severe Parkinson seen only in chronic HE
Sleep latency, sleep fragmentation, inversion of sleep-wake pattern	Impaired hydroxylation and sulfation to 6-sulfatoxymelatonin in the liver[26] Ammonia levels[27]	—

(continued on next page)

Table 2 (continued)		
Symptom	Cause	Comments
Fetor hepaticus	Attributed to dimethyl sulfide, a volatile sulfur compound that can be identified in the breath and serum of patients with cirrhosis[28]	Found in cirrhotics with or without HE
Hyperventilation	Associated with acidotic pH: compensatory mechanism that decreases the entrance of ammonia into the brain	It has also been related to increased levels of estrogens and progesterone[29]
Hepatic dementia	Pathogenetic mechanism is obscure Associated neuronal loss	In chronic HE Fluctuating symptoms with periods of improvement and a subcortical pattern The initial manifestations are attention deficits, visuopractic abnormalities, dysarthria, and apraxia Seen rarely; is reversible after LT/TIPS[30]
Hepatic parkinsonism	Pathogenetic mechanism is obscure Associated demyelination along the pyramidal tract	In chronic HE Resembles Parkinson disease, except for a symmetric presentation and lack of significant tremor
Hepatic myelopathy	Pathogenetic mechanism is obscure[31]	In chronic HE Usually motor abnormalities exceed mental deterioration Is characterized by a progressive spastic paraparesis accompanied by hyperreflexia and extensor plantar responses Only a few patients have sensory symptoms or incontinence Does not respond to standard therapy

Abbreviations: GABA, gamma-aminobutyric acid; LT, liver transplant; TIPS, transjugular intrahepatic portosystemic shunt.

DIFFERENTIAL DIAGNOSIS OF HEPATIC ENCEPHALOPATHY

Distinguishing HE from other causes of altered mental status changes may be challenging in cirrhotics[8] (**Box 1**).

SLEEP DISTURBANCE

Insomnia and hypersomnia are common early manifestations of HE. 50% to 65% of patients with cirrhosis complain of unsatisfactory sleep, with both increased sleep latency and excessive sleep fragmentation.[5,6,37,38] Sleep disturbances with cirrhosis or

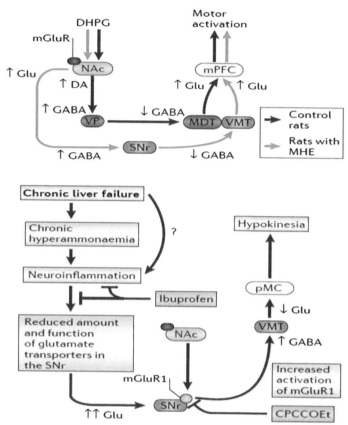

Fig. 3. Mechanism of the motor manifestations of MHE. DA, dopamine; DHPG, 3,5-dihydrox-yphenylglycine; mPFC, medial prefrontal cortex; pMC, primary motor cortex; SNr, substantia nigra pars reticulata; VMT, ventromedial thalamus; VP, ventral pallidum. (*From* Felipo V. Hepatic encephalopathy: effects of liver failure on brain function. Nat Rev Neurosci 2013;14(12):851–8; with permission.)

compensated liver failure (with or without HE) are more common than any other organ dysfunction.[5] The concentration of melatonin is inversely proportional to the pineal gland serotonin *N*-acetyltransferase activity with light exposure.[39] In chronic liver disease, the melatonin metabolism (hydroxylation and sulfation) to 6-sulfatoxymelatonin (aMT6s) is adversely affected, resulting in increased aMT6s in the urine.[40,41]

CAPACITY TO DRIVE

Psychomotor coordination, audiovisual perception, attention, and cognition all play a vital role in safe driving.[42] MHE is characterized by defects in visuospatial assessment, attention span, working memory, and speed of information processing and motor abilities.[43] Diminished driving ability in these patients has been shown[44]; psychometric testing has indicated that between 15% and 75% of patients with MHE were unable to safely drive a motor vehicle.[45,46] A pilot study of stable individuals with cirrhosis found that although 66% of the subjects had MHE, they did not show major

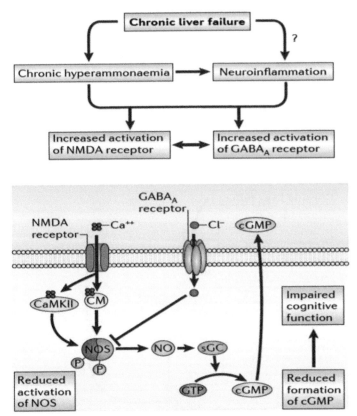

Fig. 4. Mechanism of cognitive impairment in MHE. CaMKII, calcium/calmodulin-dependent protein kinase II; GABA$_A$, type A GABA; NMDA, N-methyl-D-aspartate receptor; NO, nitric oxide; NOS, neuronal NO synthase; P, phosphorylates; sGC, soluble guanylyl cyclase. (*From* Felipo V. Hepatic encephalopathy: effects of liver failure on brain function. Nat Rev Neurosci 2013;14(12):851–8; with permission.)

impairments in their fitness to drive.[47] Despite significant driving deficits, patients with HE overestimate their driving abilities. The presence of MHE does not necessarily predict driving unfitness, and computer-based testing cannot reliably predict driving fitness.[48] A precise test or frequency of testing with which to identify patients at risk for driving remains uncertain. Also, the legislation for driving abilities varies from state to state in the United States. Assessment for high-risk patients (suggestions by relatives, Child-Pugh class B or C, large portal-systemic shunts, alcoholic liver disease, or prior episodes of HE) could be performed in which neuropsychiatric testing is available. Standardized driving tests or restrictions to daytime driving could be advised on an individual basis.[49]

In summary, physicians should follow local laws and educate patients and family of potential impairment. If possible, physicians should recommend a fitness-to-drive evaluation by an instructor trained to detect driving impairment. The driving agencies (Department of Motor Vehicles) have the ultimate authority to determine the fitness to drive. More details on driving ability and HE, including the state laws, are provided elsewhere in this issue.

> **Box 1**
> **Differential diagnosis of HE**
>
> *Overt HE or acute confusional state*
>
> Diabetic (hypoglycemia, ketoacidosis, hyperosmolar, lactate acidosis)
>
> Alcohol (intoxication, withdrawal, Wernicke)
>
> Drugs (benzodiazepines, neuroleptics, opioids)
>
> Neuroinfections
>
> Electrolyte disorders (hyponatremia and hypercalcemia)
>
> Nonconvulsive epilepsy
>
> Psychiatric disorders
>
> Intracranial bleeding and stroke
>
> Severe medical stress (organ failure and inflammation)
>
> *Other presentations*
>
> Dementia (primary and secondary)
>
> Brain lesions (traumatic, neoplasms, normal pressure hydrocephalus)
>
> Obstructive sleep apnea
>
> Hyponatremia and sepsis can both produce encephalopathy per se and precipitate HE by interactions with the pathophysiologic mechanisms. In end-stage liver disease, uremic encephalopathy and HE may overlap.
>
> *From* American Association for the Study of Liver Diseases, European Association for the Study of the Liver. Hepatic encephalopathy in chronic liver disease: 2014 practice guideline by the European Association for the Study of the Liver and the American Association for the Study of Liver Diseases. J Hepatol 2014;61(3):646; with permission.

SUMMARY

HE is a multidimensional dysfunction with several cognitive and neuropsychiatric components. A combined effort with neuropsychological and psychometric evaluation has to be performed to recognize the syndrome. MHE is largely unrecognized.

The diagnosis of HE is made through exclusion of other causes of brain dysfunction. According to the combined American Association for the Study of Liver Diseases and European Association for the Study of the Liver guidelines released in December 2014, OHE should be diagnosed by clinical criteria and can be graded according to the West Haven Criteria (the gold standard) and the Glasgow Coma Scale. The diagnosis of MHE can be made by experienced examiners using several neurophysiologic and psychometric tests. There is now a simpler smartphone application (Stroop) which is a short and valid method to screen MHE.

The clinical manifestations of HE frequently recur despite treatment, and following liver transplantation some mental deficits persists permanently.[50] Even patients with normal psychometric tests should be followed every 6 months with repeated examinations. The monitoring of neurologic symptoms needs to be dynamic, and patients with persistent HE need prompt evaluation for precipitants and adjustment of their treatment. Early diagnoses through increased awareness and evaluating the clinical manifestations would decrease the current cost burden of hospitalization (approximately US$1 billion in the United States in 2003)[51,52] for patients with OHE.

Further research to gain better insight into the pathophysiology and diagnostic accuracy of HE will help to determine future management strategies.

REFERENCES

1. Ferenci P, Lockwood A, Mullen K, et al. Hepatic encephalopathy—definition, nomenclature, diagnosis, and quantification: final report of the working party at the 11th World Congresses of Gastroenterology, Vienna, 1998. Hepatology 2002;35(3):716–21.
2. Wiltfang J, Nolte W, Weissenborn K, et al. Psychiatric aspects of portal-systemic encephalopathy. Metab Brain Dis 1998;13:379–89.
3. Weissenborn K. Diagnosis of encephalopathy. Digestion 1998;59:22–4.
4. Montagnese S, De Pitta C, De Rui M, et al. Sleep-wake abnormalities in patients with cirrhosis. Hepatology 2014;59:705–12.
5. Cordoba J, Cabrera J, Lataif L, et al. High prevalence of sleep disturbance in cirrhosis. Hepatology 1998;27:339–45.
6. Montagnese S, Middleton B, Skene DJ, et al. Night-time sleep disturbance does not correlate with neuropsychiatric impairment in patients with cirrhosis. Liver Int 2009;29:1372–82.
7. Basu P, Shah NJ, Farhat S, et al. Restless leg syndrome (RLS) is associated with hepatic encephalopathy (HE) in decompensated cirrhosis: a clinical pilot study. Am J Gastroenterol 2013;108(S1):144.
8. American Association for the Study of Liver Diseases, European Association for the Study of the Liver. Hepatic encephalopathy in chronic liver disease: 2014 practice guideline by the European Association for the Study of the Liver and the American Association for the Study of Liver Diseases. J Hepatol 2014; 61(3):642–59.
9. Bass NM, Mullen KD, Sanyal A, et al. Rifaximin treatment in hepatic encephalopathy. N Engl J Med 2010;362(12):1071–81.
10. Bajaj JS. Minimal hepatic encephalopathy matters in daily life. World J Gastroenterol 2008;14(23):3609–15.
11. Seyan AS, Hughes RD, Shawcross DL. Changing face of hepatic encephalopathy: role of inflammation and oxidative stress. World J Gastroenterol 2010;16(27):3347–57.
12. Bajaj JS, Wade JB, Sanyal AJ. Spectrum of neurocognitive impairment in cirrhosis: implications for the assessment of hepatic encephalopathy. Hepatology 2009;50:2014–21.
13. Hermenegildo C, Marcaida G, Montoliu C, et al. NMDA receptor antagonists prevent acute ammonia toxicity in mice. Neurochem Res 1996;21:1237–44.
14. Felipo V. Nature reviews. Neuroscience 2013;14:851–8.
15. Ahboucha S, Butterworth RF. Pathophysiology of hepatic encephalopathy: a new look at GABA from the molecular standpoint. Metab Brain Dis 2004;19(3–4):331–43.
16. Blei AT. Infection, inflammation and hepatic encephalopathy, synergism redefined. J Hepatol 2004;40(2):327–30.
17. Dam G, Keiding S, Munk OL, et al. Hepatic encephalopathy is associated with decreased cerebral oxygen metabolism and blood flow, not increased ammonia uptake. Hepatology 2013;57(1):258–65.
18. Häussinger D, Kircheis G, Fischer R, et al. Hepatic encephalopathy in chronic liver disease: a clinical manifestation of astrocyte swelling and low-grade cerebral edema? J Hepatol 2000;32(6):1035–8.
19. Albrecht J, Norenberg MD. Glutamine: a Trojan horse in ammonia neurotoxicity. Hepatology 2006;44:788–94.
20. Cadranel JF, Lebiez E, Di Martino V, et al. Focal neurological signs in hepatic encephalopathy in cirrhotic patients: an underestimated entity? Am J Gastroenterol 2001;96:515–8.

21. Delanty N, French JA, Labar DR, et al. Status epilepticus arising de novo in hospitalized patients: an analysis of 41 patients. Seizure 2001;10:116–9.
22. Timmermann L, Gross J, Butz M, et al. Mini-asterixis in hepatic encephalopathy induced by pathologic thalamo-motor-cortical coupling. Neurology 2003;61(5): 689–92.
23. Adams RD, Foley JM. The neurological changes in the more common types of severe liver disease. Trans Am Neurol Assoc 1949;74:217–9.
24. Krieger D, Krieger S, Jansen O, et al. Manganese and chronic hepatic encephalopathy. Lancet 1995;346:270–4.
25. Talwalkar JA, Kamath PS. influence of recent advances in medical management on clinical outcomes of cirrhosis. Mayo Clin Proc 2005;80:1501–8.
26. Boutin JA, Audinot V, Ferry G, et al. Molecular tools to study melatonin pathways and actions. Trends Pharmacol Sci 2005;26:412–9.
27. Kurtz D, Zenglein JP, Imler M, et al. Night sleep in porto-caval encephalopathy. Electroencephalogr Clin Neurophysiol 1972;33:167–78 [in French].
28. Nolte W, Wiltfang J, Schindler CG, et al. Bright basal ganglia in T1-weighted magnetic resonance images are frequent in patients with portal vein thrombosis without liver cirrhosis and not suggestive of hepatic encephalopathy. J Hepatol 1998;29(3):443–9.
29. Lustik SJ, Chhibber AK, Kolano JW, et al. The hyperventilation of cirrhosis: progesterone and estradiol effects. Hepatology 1997;25(1):55–8.
30. Larsen FS, Ranek L, Hansen BA, et al. Chronic portosystemic hepatic encephalopathy refractory to medical treatment successfully reversed by liver transplantation. Transpl Int 1995;8(3):246–7.
31. Mendoza G, Marti-Fabregas J, Kulisevsky J, et al. Hepatic myelopathy: a rare complication of portacaval shunt. Eur Neurol 1994;34(4):209–12.
32. Victor M, Adams RD, Cole M. The acquired (non Wilsonian) type of chronic hepatocerebral degeneration. Medicine 1965;44:345–96.
33. Tryc AB, Goldbecker A, Berding G, et al. Cirrhosis-related Parkinsonism: prevalence, mechanisms and response to treatments. J Hepatol 2013;58: 698–705.
34. Monfort P, Muñoz MD, ElAyadi A, et al. Effects of hyperammonemia and liver disease on glutamatergic neurotransmission. Metab Brain Dis 2002;17:237–50.
35. Cauli O, Rodrigo R, Llansola M, et al. Glutamatergic and gabaergic neurotransmission and neuronal circuits in hepatic encephalopathy. Metab Brain Dis 2009; 24:69–80.
36. Shawcross DL, Davies NA, Williams R, et al. Systemic inflammatory response exacerbates the neuropsychological effects of induced hyperammonemia in cirrhosis. J Hepatol 2004;40:247–54.
37. Bianchi G, Marchesini G, Nicolino F, et al. Psychological status and depression in patients with liver cirrhosis. Dig Liver Dis 2005;37:593–600.
38. Mostacci B, Ferlisi M, Baldi AA, et al. Sleep disturbance and daytime sleepiness in patients with cirrhosis: a case control study. Neurol Sci 2008;29:237–40.
39. Arendt J. Light-dark control of melatonin synthesis. Melatonin and the mammalian pineal gland. 1st edition. London: Chapman & Hall; 1995. p. 66–109.
40. Steindl PE, Finn B, Bendok B, et al. Disruption of the diurnal rhythm of plasma melatonin in cirrhosis. Ann Intern Med 1995;123:274–7.
41. Steindl PE, Ferenci P, Marktl W. Impaired hepatic catabolism of melatonin in cirrhosis. Ann Intern Med 1997;127:494.
42. Marshall SC. The role of reduced fitness to drive due to medical impairments in explaining crashes involving older drivers. Traffic Inj Prev 2008;9:291–8.

43. Quero JC, Schalm SW. Subclinical hepatic encephalopathy. Semin Liver Dis 1996;16:321–8.

44. Bajaj JS. Minimal hepatic encephalopathy is associated with motor vehicle crashes: the reality beyond the driving test. Hepatology 2009;50(4):1175–83.

45. Schomerus H, Hamster W, Blunck H, et al. Latent portosystemic encephalopathy. Nature of cerebral function defects and their effect on fitness to drive. Dig Dis Sci 1981;16:321–8.

46. Haussinger D, Schliess F. Pathogenetic mechanisms of hepatic encephalopathy. Gut 2008;57:1156–65.

47. Srivastava A, Mehta R, Rothke SP, et al. Fitness to drive in patients with cirrhosis and portal-systemic shunting: a pilot study evaluating driving performance. J Hepatol 1994;21(6):1023.

48. Kircheis G, Knoche A, Hilger N, et al. Hepatic encephalopathy and fitness to drive. Gastroenterology 2009;137(5):1706.

49. Córdoba J, Lucke R. Driving under the influence of minimal hepatic encephalopathy. Hepatology 2004;39(3):599.

50. Garcia-Martinez R, Rovira A, Alonso J, et al. Hepatic encephalopathy is associated with posttransplant cognitive function and brain volume. Liver Transpl 2011;17:38–46.

51. Stepanova M, Mishra A, Venkatesan C, et al. In-hospital mortality and economic burden associated with hepatic encephalopathy in the United States from 2005 to 2009. Clin Gastroenterol Hepatol 2012;10:1034–41.

52. Poorad FF. Review article: the burden of hepatic encephalopathy. Aliment Pharmacol Ther 2007;25(Suppl 1):3–9.

Covert Hepatic Encephalopathy
Who Should Be Tested and Treated?

Steven L. Flamm, MD

KEYWORDS

- Minimal hepatic encephalopathy • Covert hepatic encephalopathy • Rifaximin
- Probiotics • Encephalapp stroop test • Psychometric hepatic encephalopathy score
- Inhibitory control test • Critical flicker frequency

KEY POINTS

- Covert hepatic encephalopathy (CHE) is a common problem in the cirrhotic population, affecting up to 80%.
- Although it is not diagnosed clinically, it is a serious issue that has shown an increased risk of developing overt hepatic encephalopathy and is independently associated with poor survival and an increased risk of hospitalization.
- The clinical issues complicating CHE include diminished quality of life and work productivity and attention deficits that lead to poor driving performance.
- Rifaximin and probiotics have shown promise for the treatment of CHE.

Covert hepatic encephalopathy (CHE) is an enigmatic complication of portal hypertension. Because it is difficult to diagnose and the manifestations are subtle, CHE has often been ignored. However, emerging data suggest that the ramifications of CHE are substantial and treatment may be beneficial. This article discusses the background and clinical consequences of CHE, diagnostic strategies, and emerging data regarding therapy.

BACKGROUND

Minimal hepatic encephalopathy (MHE), formerly called *subclinical encephalopathy*, and CHE are composed of test-dependent brain dysfunction with clinical consequences in the setting of patients with chronic liver disease who are not disoriented.[1] Minimal encephalopathy indicates that there are no obvious clinical signs of

The author has nothing to disclose.
Liver Transplantation Program, Northwestern Feinberg School of Medicine, Arkes 19-041, 676 North Saint Clair, Chicago, IL 60611, USA
E-mail address: s-flamm@northwestern.edu

encephalopathy. However, as data have accumulated about the impact of minimal encephalopathy on many facets of every day life, it is clear that this term does not accurately describe the entity. The term *CHE*, which includes minimal encephalopathy and grade 1 overt hepatic encephalopathy (OHE), has been adopted (**Table 1**).[1]

CHE is observed within the spectrum of hepatic encephalopathy (HE). It is characterized by abnormalities in central nervous function with impairment in attention, psychomotor speed, visuospatial perception and delayed information processing.[2–5] It differs from OHE in that CHE, by definition, is not confirmed clinically. Specialized testing to identify patients with CHE is required.[1,2] CHE has often been ignored as an important entity because it is difficult to diagnose; there is a notion that if the manifestations are difficult to perceive, it must not be important. However, it is clear that patients with CHE have impaired quality of life (QOL), poor work productivity, and issues with driving.[6–14] Furthermore, the risk of development of OHE is augmented; there is increased associated mortality and a risk of hospitalization.[15–17]

Because CHE is so common in cirrhosis, affecting up to 80% of patients, more interest has arisen in this entity in recent years.[18–21]

DIAGNOSIS

There has been reluctance to perform a diagnostic work-up for CHE for diverse reasons. First, there is a lack of awareness about the problem because it is often not discussed and because the clinical consequences are difficult to observe. Further, the diagnostic tests are somewhat obscure. The lack of standardization of a definitive diagnostic testing regimen has also hindered widespread usage of the tests to diagnose CHE.

Before conferring a diagnosis of CHE, other causes of impaired mentation, such as ischemic neurologic injury, metabolic abnormalities, dementia, or medication-induced cognitive impairment, must be ruled out. Initial evaluation should include eliciting a careful history including prescription medications, over-the-counter products, and usage of alcohol and/or illicit drugs. A neurologic examination should be performed. Finally, the Mini-Mental State Examination (MMSE), a simple test that assesses basic cognitive function and is a screening test for dementia, should be administered.[22] If

Table 1 MHE and CHE		Description	Manifestation
Minimal	Covert	Psychometric or neuropsychological alterations of tests exploring psychomotor speed/executive functions or neurophysiological alterations without clinical evidence of mental change	There are abnormal results of established psychometric or neuropsychological tests without clinical manifestations.
Grade 1		Trivial lack of awareness Euphoria or anxiety Shortened attention span Impairment of addition or subtraction Altered sleep rhythm	Despite oriented in time and space, patients seem to have some cognitive/behavioral decay with respect to their standard on clinical examination or to the caregivers.

Modified from Vilstrup H, Amodio P, Bajaj J, et al. Hepatic encephalopathy in chronic liver disease: 2014 practice guideline by the European Association for the Study of the Liver and the American Association for the Study of Liver Diseases. Hepatology 2014;60(2):715–35.

the MMSE is normal and if another diagnosis is not suspected, CHE remains a possibility.

Many diagnostic tests have been evaluated to diagnose CHE.[23,24]

Venous Ammonia Levels

Serum venous ammonia levels have not been helpful in the diagnosis of CHE because the level is affected by many extraneous factors and does not correlate with neurologic dysfunction.[1,25]

Psychometric Tests

Several psychometric tests have been implemented for the diagnosis of CHE, designed to identify deficits in attention, response time and inhibition, and visuospatial function. Some are pencil-and-paper tests, whereas others are computerized. The following discussion includes commonly used psychometric tests but is not all inclusive (**Table 2**).[26]

Psychometric hepatic encephalopathy score

The current recommended battery of tests that was developed and validated for diagnosis of CHE is composed of 5 psychometric tests that yields the Psychometric Hepatic Encephalopathy Score (PHES).[26,27] It was endorsed by the Working Party at the 11th World Congress of Gastroenterology.[18] The tests include the number connection tests A and B (NCT-A and NCT-B), the digit symbol test (DST), the serial dotting test, and the line-tracing test. It should be noted that the PHES is copyrighted and has not been validated in the United States.[28]

If the PHES cannot be completed in its entirety, the Working Group endorsed 4 tests for diagnosing CHE, the NCT-A, NCT-B, DST, and the block design test. Abnormalities in 2 of the tests (at least 2 standard deviations from age- and education-matched controls) would identify CHE.

Although the battery is easy to administer, it is somewhat time consuming and difficult to interpret; it is infrequently available to practicing clinicians, limiting general applicability of the PHES. In addition, because there is a learning component of the tests, repeatability is an issue. Plus one must have fine motor skills because the tests are carried out with pencil and paper.

Repeatable battery for the assessment of neurologic status

An alternative to PHES is the Repeatable Battery for the Assessment of Neurologic Status (RBANS; Pearson Education, Inc, San Antonio, TX, USA) and has been recommended for diagnosis of CHE by the International Society for the Study of Hepatic Encephalopathy and Nitrogen Metabolism.[27] RBANS is also copyrighted.[28] It has identified CHE in several studies.[29,30] The test has 2 domains, cortical and subcortical. The applicability of RBANS in practice is limited because it must be administered and scored by a psychologist.

Inhibitory control test

Another technique that has been trumpeted for diagnosis of CHE is the computerized Inhibitory Control Test (ICT).[31] ICT assesses response inhibition and attention, with particular emphasis on visuomotor function and reaction time. The test consists of series of random letters crossing over a computer screen with a target letter combination and lures of false letter combinations. Patients are evaluated on correct response to targets, incorrect responses to lures, and reaction times.[23] ICT is easy to administer and scoring is automated, highlighting its potential utility in clinical practice.

Table 2
Common diagnostic tests for chronic HE

Type	Test	Description
Pencil-and-paper tests	PHES	Includes 5 tests: NCT-A and NCT-B (concentration, mental tracking, and visuomotor speed), line tracing (visuomotor and visuospatial speed and accuracy), serial dotting (psychomotor speed), and digit symbol (psychomotor and visuomotor speed) tests
	RBANS (Pearson Education, Inc, San Antonio, TX, USA)	Measures of verbal and visual memory, working memory, cognitive processing speed, language, and visuospatial function (ie, line orientation and figure copy); there are 4 alternate forms (A–D) US population-based standardization for patients aged 20–89 y and generates age-scaled index scores with a normal mean of 100
Computerized tests	ICT	Test of attention and response inhibition that consists of presentation of letters at 500-ms intervals; interspersed within these letters are the letters X and Y Patients instructed to respond only when X and Y are alternating (targets) and to refrain from responding when X and Y are not alternating (lures) Requires a training run and 6 test runs (lasting ~2 min each), for a total of 40 lures, 212 targets, and 1726 random letters in between
	Stroop	Stroop tasks used to evaluate psychomotor speed and cognitive flexibility; now available as a smartphone application Includes an off state with symbols only (no words); must correctly and rapidly press the color corresponding to the color of the symbols presented Includes an on state with words in discordant colors; must correctly and rapidly press the color corresponding to the color of the word presented, not the color it means 10 stimuli in each run; stops after one mistake; need 5 complete runs in off-and-on state; measures the number of runs needed to achieve 5 correct runs and the time needed to complete those 5 correct runs
Neurologic tests	CFF	Tests patients' reaction time by evaluating the ability of a patient to perceive flickering light; based on principle that retinal glial cells in patients with HE undergo similar changes (eg, swelling) to those in cerebral glial cells Must identify frequency at which a flickering light perceived as continuous at first begins to be perceived intermittently as the flickering frequency decreases
	Electroencephalogram/evoked potentials	Measures and records electrical brain activity

Abbreviations: NCT-A, number connection test A; NCT-B, number connection test B.
Modified from Kappus MR, Bajaj JS. Assessment of minimal hepatic encephalopathy (with emphasis on computerized psychometric tests). Clin Liver Dis 2012;16:43–55.

Smartphone application

Stroop tasks measure psychomotor speed and cognitive flexibility and have been validated for the diagnosis of CHE.[32] It consists of identifying the color of symbols presented, delineating the correct color of a color word that is a different color than the word itself (eg, *red* in a green-colored font), and reaction times. This test is easy to administer and grade and is readily available. However, it requires a smartphone and download of the application through the Apple Store (Apple Inc, Cupertino, CA, USA).

Neurophysiologic Tests

Other diagnostic strategies have been implemented that have a neurophysiologic basis.

Critical flicker frequency

In the research setting, the critical flicker frequency (CFF) test, a test of cortical function, has been used.[33–36] A light impulse is presented to patients, oscillating at a frequency of 60 Hz. This impulse is perceived as a constant dot of light. The frequency is then decreased steadily until patients detect the light as a flicker. Patients with CHE perceive the flicker at a lower frequency than patients who do not.[23] The test has been useful elsewhere, although it has not been validated in the United States. Although CFF is easy to perform and is inexpensive, special equipment is required that is not easy to obtain or repair.

Electroencephalogram

The electroencephalogram (EEG) is another test that has been used within the context of research studies in the setting of HE.[37–40] Although rhythm slowing is observed in HE, definitive specific abnormalities for CHE have not been identified. Evoked potentials, the time between a stimulus and the sensation of it by the brain, have also been investigated. Differences in visual and auditory evoked late potentials (P300) have been observed in patients with CHE.[38,40,41]

EEG and evoked potentials to date have not been shown to provide diagnostic information critical for the diagnosis of CHE. The testing is time consuming, expensive, and requires trained personnel. At present, there is little role for EEG and evoked potentials outside of the research setting in CHE.

Imaging Modalities

Imaging modalities, such as head MRI, magnetic resonance spectroscopy, single-photon emission computed tomography, and PET, have also shown various changes in patients with CHE.[42–45] However, the tests are expensive and nonspecific for CHE; therefore, general use for diagnosis of CHE is impractical.

CLINICAL MANIFESTATIONS

Patients with CHE do not have verbal deficits, suggesting that it is not an important problem. However, substantial decrements in QOL and diminished work productivity are the rule.[6–10] In addition, patients with CHE have impaired driving ability and have more traffic accidents than matched controls.[11–14] The deficits responsible for these issues are under the umbrella of impaired attention. Affected patients have difficulties with orientation and vigilance. Higher executive functions, such as working memory and ability to learn, are also decreased.

Thus, CHE has widespread unfavorable effects on patients' lives.

TREATMENT

Because the clinical manifestations of CHE are subtle and the diagnostic tests are somewhat obscure and not standardized, treatment has largely been restricted to clinical trials. Several strategies have been successful (**Box 1**).

Nonabsorbable Disaccharides

Lactulose and lactitol are nonabsorbable disaccharides. They are used to treat OHE; such products are thought to work by increasing excretion of gut-derived toxins, such as ammonia, by augmenting colonic transit and perhaps by decreasing colon luminal pH.[21,23] These products are poorly tolerated, with nausea, flatus, abdominal cramps, and diarrhea as frequent side effects. Nevertheless, lactulose/lactitol have been examined in several trials in the treatment of CHE.[46–50] In one study involving 61 patients, lactulose at a dosage of 30 to 60 mL daily over 3 months in 31 subjects was found to significantly decrease the number of baseline abnormal psychometric tests compared with 30 individuals who received no treatment. A total of 64.5% of patients who received lactulose improved compared with 6.7% who received placebo.[46] Lactulose also afforded clinical benefit as a significantly greater number of patients achieved health-related QOL (HRQOL) benefit compared with no treatment. A meta-analysis of 5 studies confirmed improvement with lactulose therapy compared with no treatment.[51]

Unfortunately, because of the poor tolerance for lactulose leading to decreased compliance and the subtle clinical manifestations that CHE presents, it is unlikely that lactulose will gain widespread acceptance for CHE in community practice, either from patients or from health care practitioners.

Antibiotics

Antibiotics have been used for many years in the treatment of OHE. The proposed mechanism of action is reduction or elimination of urease-producing intestinal bacteria that are responsible for the production of ammonia and other gut-derived toxins that cause OHE.[23,52,53] In the past, antibiotics have been used in patients with OHE who are refractory to lactulose or who are lactulose intolerant.

Over the years, neomycin, metronidazole, and, to a lesser extent, oral vancomycin have been administered. Unfortunately, these medications have been largely ineffective for the treatment of OHE and have been associated with systemic toxicity. Nephrotoxicity and ototoxicity may be observed with the aminoglycoside neomycin, and neurotoxicity and nausea are seen with metronidazole.[26] Usage of these agents has fallen out of favor in recent years.

Box 1
Medication class
Nonabsorbable disaccharides
Lactulose
Lactitol
Antibiotics
Rifaximin
Probiotics

Rifaximin is a minimally absorbed antibiotic that has been used for treatment of traveler's diarrhea for many years.[54] It has broad-spectrum antimicrobial activity and is thought to work by diminishing production of intestinal bacteria-derived toxins. Because absorption is minimal, and the medication is well tolerated, requiring no dose reduction in patients with renal or liver dysfunction, rifaximin offers a favorable profile for potential long-term.[55] In addition, it does not seem to alter the normal fecal flora and, thus, is not associated with *Clostridium difficile* colitis.[56–58]

The Food and Drug Administration approved rifaximin in 2010 for the prevention of the recurrence of OHE in high-risk patients. Rifaximin has also been assessed in studies for the treatment of CHE. The RIME trial was a placebo-controlled randomized double-blind trial that compared rifaximin with placebo in patients with CHE.[59] Forty-nine patients were administered rifaximin at a dosage of 1200 mg daily compared with 45 who received placebo for 8 weeks. Patients in the rifaximin group had a significantly increased improvement in CHE compared with placebo at weeks 2 and 8 and a significantly improved HRQOL at week 8 compared with baseline. Furthermore, HRQOL improvements also correlated with neuropsychometric scores at week 8.

Bajaj and colleagues[60] also examined the effects of rifaximin versus placebo on one of the adverse clinical outcomes of CHE, driving ability. The study was a placebo-controlled randomized double-blind trial that compared 21 patients who received rifaximin 550 mg and 21 subjects who received placebo, each twice daily, for 8 weeks in patients with CHE. Many outcome measures were assessed, including driving performance as determined by a driving simulator, psychometric test performance, HRQOL, cytokine levels (interleukin 10 [IL-10]), and tolerability. Driving performance was significantly improved in the rifaximin group compared with placebo at week 8. Neuropsychometric test results significantly improved more frequently in the rifaximin group (91%) compared with the placebo group (61%). Overall HRQOL did not improve by week 8 in either group. IL-10 levels were also significantly higher in the rifaximin group, with no change in the placebo group. Rifaximin was well tolerated.

Although additional studies must be performed to confirm these results, the usage of rifaximin is promising in the treatment of CHE.

Probiotics

Probiotics alter the intestinal microbiome and are thought to have putative favorable effects for encephalopathy by changing the composition of gut bacteria such that intestinal-derived toxins like ammonia are produced at lower levels.[61] Usage of probiotics has been limited because there are many different preparations and each is composed of different bacteria. Further, quality control of production of individual lots is often not as rigorous as it is for medications because probiotics are not subject to the same oversight. Nevertheless, probiotics have been assessed in the treatment of CHE in several studies.[61–66]

One study involving 105 patients randomized 35 patients to a probiotic, 35 patients to lactulose, and 35 patients to both for 1 month.[64] A similar benefit was observed in all 3 groups (51.6%–56.6%) as determined by neuropsychometric testing and auditory evoked potentials.

A second study compared 17 patients with MHE who received probiotic yogurt to 8 patients who did not for 60 days.[65] Improvement in CHE was observed in 70.6% of patients who received the probiotic yogurt versus none of the controls (highly statistically significant). However, HRQOL as measured by the 36-Item Short Form Health Survey did not improve in either group.

Another randomized study involved 35 patients with CHE; 20 patients received probiotics/fiber and 15 received placebo for 30 days.[66] The patients who received probiotics/fiber were much more likely than the patients who received placebo to reverse symptoms of CHE (50.0% vs 13.3%, respectively). In addition, there were significant decrements in serum endotoxin and venous ammonia levels in the probiotic/fiber group, and there were no differences in the placebo group.

Probiotics are promising for the treatment of CHE. However, the composition of the products must be clearly defined and production must be carefully regulated to ensure consistency. Furthermore, additional studies must be performed to define and confirm a potential benefit in the CHE population.

SHOULD WE TEST FOR COVERT HEPATIC ENCEPHALOPATHY AND, IF SO, IN WHOM?

CHE is a condition that has significant consequences that are underappreciated. In order to advocate screening patients for CHE, a definitive diagnostic testing strategy that is available, feasible, and inexpensive must be agreed on and endorsed. Further, a treatment approach should also be available and accepted once the diagnosis is made.

Because the tests to diagnose CHE are somewhat obscure and there has been delayed agreement on a definitive set of diagnostic tests, the quest to confirm CHE has not gained traction in the clinical community. There is enough information available that it would be wise for providers who care for patients with cirrhosis to pursue a more aggressive approach.

Although some have proposed screening for CHE in all cirrhotic patients, that may be unnecessary.[28,67] On the other hand, cirrhotic patients who seem to have declining QOL and/or work productivity, complain of poor short-term memory and concentration, or who have high-risk occupations (such as truck or bus drivers, airline pilots, heavy equipment operators) should be considered candidates for assessment.[19,68] In addition, patients who have other complaints suggestive of attention deficit issues should also be considered for examination. The recent American Association for the Study of Liver Diseases (AASLD)/European Association for the Study of the Liver (EASL) guidelines have recommended consideration of testing in patients who might benefit from testing, such as those with impaired QOL or in whom there are potential implications regarding public safety or employment.[1]

A diagnostic strategy of performing psychometric tests (PHES or RBANS) should be considered. Other feasible approaches include the ICT (computerized) or the EncephalApp Stroop (smartphone) tests, performed on a periodic basis in appropriate patients. The AASLD/EASL guidelines have recommended at least 2 of the currently validated testing strategies: PHES and either one of the computerized or neurophysiological testing techniques.[1]

Additional research should be pursued to outline a rational and feasible strategy that can be implemented by clinical practitioners and that is accurate for the diagnosis of CHE.

TREATMENT STRATEGIES

Additional research is necessary to define effective therapies for CHE. Probiotics are promising, but there is as of yet insufficient evidence to support recommendation of usage of probiotics for CHE. Investigation in the future should take into account a clear description of the content of the preparations so that reproducibility of the results is assured.

Lactulose has also been effective for CHE. However, lactulose is poorly tolerated and is unlikely to gain acceptance for this condition by patients or health care providers.

Regarding rifaximin, more data are necessary to confirm a favorable effect. However, data have already emerged that suggest rifaximin is a reasonable alternative in patients with CHE and should be considered if the condition is diagnosed on an individual basis.

In general, the recent AASLD/EASL guidelines have indicated that treatment of CHE should not be routinely recommended but rather should be considered on a case-by-case basis.[1]

SUMMARY

CHE is a common problem in the cirrhotic population, affecting up to 80%. Although it is not diagnosed clinically, it is a serious issue that has shown an increased risk of developing OHE and is independently associated with poor survival and an increased risk of hospitalization. The clinical issues complicating CHE are significant, including diminished QOL and work productivity and attention deficits that lead to poor driving performance. Diagnostic strategies are being honed. Psychometric tests are available in the United States. However, computerized psychometric tests, such as the ICT, the smartphone EncephalApp Stroop test, and the neurophysiologic CFF test, all offer diagnostic studies that are useful in CHE and that are feasible in clinical practice. Rifaximin and probiotics have shown promise for the treatment of CHE. Additional research must be performed to identify which cirrhotic patient groups benefit from screening and to define the appropriate screening interval. Further, more investigation must be undertaken to outline appropriate treatment strategies that are feasible for clinical practice. Finally, aggressive educational programs must be developed to communicate the importance of the consequences of CHE and how to diagnose and treat it.

ACKNOWLEDGMENTS

The author would like to thank Kristen Eis for her indispensable help in the production of this article.

REFERENCES

1. Weissenborn K, Ennen JC, Schomerus H, et al. Neuropsychological characterization of hepatic encephalopathy. J Hepatol 2001;34:768–73.
2. Schiff S, Vallesi A, Mapelli D, et al. Impairment of response inhibition precedes motor alteration in the early stage of liver cirrhosis: a behavioral electrophysiological study. Metab Brain Dis 2005;20:381–92.
3. Ortiz M, Cordoba J, Jacas C, et al. Neuropsychological abnormalities in cirrhosis include learning impairment. J Hepatol 2006;44:104–10.
4. Weissenborn K, Giewekemeyer K, Heidenreich S, et al. Attention, memory and cognitive function in hepatic encephalopathy. Metab Brain Dis 2005;20:359–67.
5. Groeneweg M, Quero JC, De Bruijn I, et al. Subclinical hepatic encephalopathy impairs daily functioning. Hepatology 1998;28:45–9.
6. Schomerus H, Hamster W. Quality of life in cirrhotics with minimal hepatic encephalopathy. Metab Brain Dis 2001;16:37–41.
7. Arguedas MR, DeLawrence TG, McGuire BM. Influence of hepatic encephalopathy on health-related quality of life in patients with cirrhosis. Dig Dis Sci 2003; 48:1622–6.
8. Bianchi G, Giovagnoli M, Sasdelli AS, et al. Hepatic encephalopathy and health-related quality of life. Clin Liver Dis 2012;16:159–70.

9. Roman E, Cordoba J, Torrens M, et al. Minimal hepatic encephalopathy is associated with falls. Am J Gastroenterol 2011;106:476–82.

10. Wein C, Koch H, Popp B, et al. Minimal hepatic encephalopathy impairs fitness to drive. Hepatology 2004;39:739–45.

11. Bajaj JS, Hafeezullah M, Hoffmann RG, et al. Minimal hepatic encephalopathy: a vehicle for accidents and traffic violations. Am J Gastroenterol 2007;102:1903–9.

12. Bajaj JS, Hafeezullah M, Hoffmann RG, et al. Navigation skill impairment: another dimension of the driving difficulties in minimal hepatic encephalopathy. Hepatology 2008;47:596–604.

13. Bajaj JS, Saeian K, Schubert CM, et al. Minimal hepatic encephalopathy is associated with motor vehicle crashes: the reality beyond the driving test. Hepatology 2009;50:1175–83.

14. Romero-Gomez M, Boza F, Garcia-Valdecasas MS, et al. Subclinical hepatic encephalopathy predicts the development of overt hepatic encephalopathy. Am J Gastroenterol 2001;96:2718–23.

15. Hartman IJ, Groeneweg M, Quero JC, et al. The prognostic significance of subclinical hepatic encephalopathy. Am J Gastroenterol 2000;95:2029–34.

16. Patidar K, Thacker L, Wade J, et al. Covert and hepatic encephalopathy is independently associated with poor survival and increased risk of hospitalization. Am J Gastroenterol 2014;109:1757–63.

17. Ferenci P, Lockwood A, Mullen K, et al. Hepatic encephalopathy – definition, nomenclature, diagnosis, and quantification. Final report of the working party at the 11th World Congresses of Gastroenterology, Vienna, 1998. Hepatology 2002;35:716–21.

18. Ortiz M, Jaccas C, Cordoba J. Minimal hepatic encephalopathy: diagnosis, clinical significance and recommendations. J Hepatol 2005;42(suppl):S45–53.

19. Li YY, Nie YQ, Sha WH, et al. Prevalence of subclinical hepatic encephalopathy in cirrhotic patients in China. World J Gastroenterol 2004;10:2397–401.

20. Blei AT, Cordoba J. Hepatic encephalopathy. Am J Gastroenterol 2001;96:1968–76.

21. Folstein MF, Folstein SE, McHugh PR. Mini-mental state: a practical method for grading the cognitive state of patients for the clinician. J Psychiatr Res 1975; 12:189–98.

22. Shawcross DL, Wright G, Olde Damink SW, et al. Role of ammonia and inflammation in minimal hepatic encephalopathy. Metab Brain Dis 2007;22:125–38.

23. Kappus MR, Bajaj JS. Assessment of minimal hepatic encephalopathy (with emphasis on computerized psychometric tests). Clin Liver Dis 2012;16(1):43–55.

24. Prakash R, Kanna S, Mullen K. Evolving concepts: the negative effect of minimal hepatic encephalopathy and role for prophylaxis in patients with cirrhosis. Clin Ther 2013;35(9):1458–73.

25. Mullen KD, Ferenci P, Bass NM, et al. An algorithm for the management of hepatic encephalopathy. Semin Liver Dis 2007;27:32–48.

26. Randolph C, Hilsabeck R, Kato A, et al. Neuropsychological assessment of hepatic encephalopathy: ISHEN practice guidelines. Liver Int 2009;29:629–35.

27. Duarte-Rojo A, Estradas J, Hernandez-Ramos R, et al. Validation of the psychometric hepatic encephalopathy score (PHES) for identifying patients with minimal hepatic encephalopathy. Dig Dis Sci 2011;56:3014–23.

28. Bajaj J. Management options for minimal hepatic encephalopathy. Expert Rev Gastroenterol Hepatol 2008;2(6):785–90.

29. Sorrell JH, Zolnikov BJ, Sharma A, et al. Cognitive impairment in people diagnosed with end-stage liver disease evaluated for liver transplantation. Psychiatry Clin Neurosci 2006;60(2):174–81.

30. Mooney S, Hassanein TI, Hilsabeck RC, et al. Utility of the Repeatable Battery for the Assessment of Neuropsychological Status (RBANS) in patients with end-stage liver disease awaiting liver transplant. Arch Clin Neuropsychol 2007;22: 175–86.
31. Bajaj JS, Hafeezullah M, Franco J, et al. Inhibitory control test for the diagnosis of minimal hepatic encephalopathy. Gastroenterology 2008;135:1591–600.
32. Bajaj JS, Thacker LR, Heuman DM, et al. The Stroop smartphone application is a short and valid method to screen for minimal hepatic encephalopathy. Hepatology 2013;58:1122–32.
33. Haussinger D, Kircheis G, Fischer R, et al. Hepatic encephalopathy in chronic liver disease: a clinical manifestation of astrocyte swelling and low grade cerebral edema. J Hepatol 2000;32:1035–8.
34. Romero-Gomez M, Cordoba J, Jover R, et al. Value of the critical flicker frequency in patients with minimal hepatic encephalopathy. Hepatology 2007;45:879–85.
35. Kircheis G, Wettstein M, Timmermann L, et al. Critical flicker frequency for quantification of low-grade hepatic encephalopathy. Hepatology 2002;35:357–66.
36. Sharma P, Sharma BC, Sarin SK. Critical flicker frequency for diagnosis and assessment of recovery from minimal hepatic encephalopathy in patients with cirrhosis. Hepatobiliary Pancreat Dis Int 2010;9:27–32.
37. Parsons-Smith BG, Summerskill WH, Dawson AM, et al. The electroencephalograph in liver disease. Lancet 1957;273:867–71.
38. Amodio P, Del Piccolo F, Petteno E, et al. Prevalence and prognostic value of quantified electroencephalogram (EEG) alterations in cirrhotic patients. J Hepatol 2001;35:37–45.
39. Montagnese S, Jackson C, Morgan MY. Spatio-temporal decomposition of the electroencephalogram in patients with cirrhosis. J Hepatol 2007;46:447–58.
40. Amodio P, Campagna F, Olianas S, et al. Detection of minimal hepatic encephalopathy: normalization and optimization of the psychometric hepatic encephalopathy score. A neuropsychological and quantified EEG study. J Hepatol 2008;49: 346–53.
41. Saxena N, Bhatia M, Joshi YK, et al. Auditory P300 event-related potentials and number connection test for evaluation of subclinical hepatic encephalopathy in patients with cirrhosis of the liver: a follow-up study. J Gastroenterol Hepatol 2001;16:322–7.
42. Weissenborn K, Ehrenheim C, Hori A, et al. Pallidal lesions in patients with liver cirrhosis: clinical and MRI evaluation. Metab Brain Dis 1995;10:219–31.
43. Naegele T, Grodd W, Viebahn R, et al. MR imaging and (1) H spectroscopy of brain metabolites in hepatic encephalopathy: time-course of renormalization after liver transplantation. Radiology 2000;216:683–91.
44. Trzepacz PT, Tarter RE, Shah A, et al. SPECT scan and cognitive findings in subclinical hepatic encephalopathy. J Neuropsychiatry Clin Neurosci 1994;6: 170–5.
45. Lockwood AH, Weissenborn K, Bokemeyer M, et al. Correlations between cerebral glucose metabolism and neuropsychological test performance in nonalcoholic cirrhotics. Metab Brain Dis 2002;17:29–40.
46. Prasad S, Dhiman RK, Duseja A, et al. Lactulose improves cognitive functions and health-related quality of life in patients with cirrhosis who have minimal hepatic encephalopathy. Hepatology 2007;45:549–59.
47. Morgan MY, Alonso M, Stanger LC. Lactitol and lactulose for the treatment of subclinical hepatic encephalopathy in cirrhotic patients. A randomised, cross-over study. J Hepatol 1989;8:208–17.

48. Watanabe A, Sakai T, Sato S, et al. Clinical efficacy of lactulose in cirrhotic patients with and without subclinical hepatic encephalopathy. Hepatology 1997; 26:1410–4.

49. Horsmans Y, Solbreux PM, Daenens C, et al. Lactulose improves psychometric testing in cirrhotic patients with subclinical encephalopathy. Aliment Pharmacol Ther 1997;11:165–70.

50. Zeng Z, Li YY. Effects of lactulose treatment on the course of subclinical hepatic encephalopathy. Zhonghua Yi Xue Za Zhi 2003;83:1126–9.

51. Shukla S, Shukla A, Mehboob S, et al. Meta-analysis: the effects of gut flora modulation using prebiotics, probiotics and synbiotics on minimal hepatic encephalopathy. Aliment Pharmacol Ther 2011;33:662–71.

52. Riordan SM, Williams R. Gut flora and hepatic encephalopathy in patients with cirrhosis. N Engl J Med 2010;362:1140–2.

53. Seyan AS, Hughes RD, Shawcross DL. Changing face of hepatic encephalopathy: role of inflammation and oxidative stress. World J Gastroenterol 2010;16: 3347–57.

54. DuPont HL, Jiang ZD, Okhuysen PC, et al. A randomized, double-blind, placebo-controlled trial of rifaximin to prevent travelers' diarrhea. Ann Intern Med 2005; 142:805–12.

55. Xifaxan (rifaximin) tablets [package insert]. Raleigh, NC: Salix Pharmaceuticals, Inc; 2012.

56. Bajaj JS, Heuman DM, Sanyal AJ, et al. Modulation of the metabiome by rifaximin in patients with cirrhosis and minimal hepatic encephalopathy. PLoS One 2013;8: e60042.

57. Brigidi P, Swennen E, Rizzello F, et al. Effects of rifaximin administration on the intestinal microbiota in patients with ulcerative colitis. J Chemother 2002;14:290–5.

58. Bass NM, Mullen KD, Sanyal A, et al. Rifaximin treatment in hepatic encephalopathy. N Engl J Med 2010;362:1071–81.

59. Sidhu SS, Goyal O, Mishra BP, et al. Rifaximin improves psychometric performance and health-related quality of life in patients with minimal hepatic encephalopathy (the RIME Trial). Am J Gastroenterol 2011;106:307–16.

60. Bajaj JS, Heuman DM, Wade JB, et al. Rifaximin improves driving simulator performance in a randomized trial of patients with minimal hepatic encephalopathy. Gastroenterology 2011;140:478–87.

61. Saji S, Kumar S, Thomas V. A randomized double blind placebo controlled trial of probiotics in minimal hepatic encephalopathy. Trop Gastroenterol 2011;32: 128–32.

62. Lata J, Jurankova J, Pribramska V, et al. Effect of administration of Escherichia coli Nissle (Mutaflor) on intestinal colonisation, endo-toxemia, liver function and minimal hepatic encephalopathy in patients with liver cirrhosis. Vnitr Lek 2006; 52:215–9.

63. Malaguarnera M, Greco F, Barone G, et al. Bifidobacterium longum with fructo-oligosaccharide (FOS) treatment in minimal hepatic encephalopathy: a randomized, double-blind, placebo-controlled study. Dig Dis Sci 2007;52:3259–65.

64. Sharma P, Sharma BC, Puri V, et al. An open-label randomized controlled trial of lactulose and probiotics in the treatment of minimal hepatic encephalopathy. Eur J Gastroenterol Hepatol 2008;20:506–11.

65. Bajaj JS, Saeian K, Christensen KM, et al. Probiotic yogurt for the treatment of minimal hepatic encephalopathy. Am J Gastroenterol 2008;103:1707–15.

66. Liu Q, Duan ZP, Ha DK, et al. Synbiotic modulation of gut flora: effect on minimal hepatic encephalopathy in patients with cirrhosis. Hepatology 2004;39:1441–9.

67. Quero Guillen JC, Groeneweg M, Jimenez SM, et al. Is it a medical error if we do not screen cirrhotic patients for minimal hepatic encephalopathy? Rev Esp Enferm Dig 2002;94:544–57.
68. Stewart CA, Smith GE. Minimal hepatic encephalopathy. Nat Clin Pract Gastroenterol Hepatol 2007;4:677–85.

Should We Treat Minimal/ Covert Hepatic Encephalopathy, and with What?

CrossMark

Phillip K. Henderson, DO[a], Jorge L. Herrera, MD[b],*

KEYWORDS

- Encephalopathy • Covert hepatic encephalopathy • Overt encephalopathy
- Minimal hepatic encephalopathy

KEY POINTS

- Despite its name, minimal hepatic encephalopathy significantly impacts quality of life and daily function.
- Most patients with cirrhosis develop covert encephalopathy during the natural history of their disease.
- Probiotics, nonabsorbable dissacharides, rifaximin, and L-ornithine-L-aspartate have all been studied for treatment of covert hepatic encephalopathy (CHE).
- Because of lack of readily accessible testing strategies, detection and treatment of CHE remains suboptimal and dependent on regional resources and expertise.

INTRODUCTION

Hepatic encephalopathy (HE) is a heterogeneous class of neuropsychiatric changes seen in cirrhosis in the absence of other organic brain disorders.[1] HE is a spectrum of neurocognitive impairments in cirrhosis that range from abnormal neuropsychiatric testing without clinical evidence of disease (minimal HE [MHE]) to varying degrees of overt clinical findings (overt HE [OHE]).[1] The categories of OHE are broken down by their cause: acute liver failure (type A), bypass (type B), and cirrhosis (type C). The West Haven classification is used to discern the varying degrees of OHE.[2] Much debate has centered on the term "minimal" in MHE because of the concern for trivialization of the neurocognitive impairment in this subgroup by patients and clinicians.[2] The term covert HE (CHE) has been adopted and accepted by the International

The authors have nothing to disclose.
[a] Division of Gastroenterology, University of South Alabama, 6000 University Commons, 75 University Boulevard South, Mobile, AL 36688, USA; [b] Division of Hepatology, University of South Alabama, 6000 University Commons, 75 University Boulevard South, Mobile, AL 36688, USA
* Corresponding author.
E-mail address: jherrera@health.southalabama.edu

Clin Liver Dis 19 (2015) 487–495
http://dx.doi.org/10.1016/j.cld.2015.04.002
1089-3261/15/$ – see front matter © 2015 Elsevier Inc. All rights reserved.

liver.theclinics.com

Society for Hepatic Encephalopathy and Nitrogen Metabolism to address this misconception.[2] CHE refers to all subclinical HE not detectable by history and physical examination, and includes minimal encephalopathy and West Haven grade I OHE.[1]

CHE is extremely common with up to 80% of patients with cirrhosis being affected.[3] Because of the lack of clinically detectable changes in verbal skills or motor function, the diagnosis of CHE is difficult and requires specialized testing to discern the subtle changes in cognition. The tools currently available for the diagnosis of CHE have been reviewed elsewhere in this issue. Some of these specialized psychometric tests require advanced training to perform and are not readily available in clinical practice. A survey of 137 members of the American Association for the Study of Liver Disease showed only 40% of the respondents routinely tested their patients for CHE. The surveyed group reported that the time and resource allocation required for diagnosis was a major barrier.[4] Because of the lack of an easily performed standardized screening tool and controversy over which patients should be screened CHE remains an underdiagnosed condition.

COVERT ENCEPHALOPATHY: IS IT IMPORTANT?

Deficits in attention and coordination that are seen in CHE affect multiple dimensions of life in a patient with cirrhosis despite not being clinically detectable. Quality of life (QOL) is impacted in patients with CHE and translated into lower QOL scores.[5] Studies by Groeneweg and colleagues[6] have shown significant impact on activities of daily living using the Sickness Impact Profile (SIP). The SIP, which has been validated across a broad range of chronic medical conditions, detects significant impacts on the QOL of patients with cirrhosis with CHE.[1] The SIP uses physical, social, and psychological domains to grade the degree of QOL impairment. The study by Groeneweg and colleagues[6] showed that patients with CHE have significantly reduced scores in all domains. The most affected areas were alertness, home management, work, recreational activities, and sleep.[3]

Falls are a significant burden to health care use and account for 90% of fracture visits in emergency departments.[7] The subclinical visual-motor impairment in patients with CHE puts them at risk for falls.[8] Falls have been shown to be more common in patients with cirrhosis with CHE than without. Patients taking concurrent psychotropic medications were further at risk for falls.[9] The increased prevalence of decreased bone mineral density among patients with cirrhosis places them at increased risk for fracture with falls. In the study by Roman and colleagues[9] one-third of patients with CHE who fell sustained a fracture and hospital stays were longer and more costly in patients with CHE compared with patients with cirrhosis without CHE and healthy control subjects. Of note, all patients who were hospitalized because of falls with CHE experienced hepatic decompensation, whereas no patients hospitalized without CHE experienced decompensation.[9]

The attention and coordination defects seen in CHE also affect the ability to work. Schomerus and Hamster[10] demonstrated that employability is affected by CHE. Blue collar workers whose employment centers on repetitive motion or manual labor are most affected by covert encephalopathy.[1] Direct financial impact comes when these patients are unable to maintain employment or perform at work. Fellow coworkers who may be injured by subclinically impaired patients and caretaker burden contribute to the indirect costs of CHE.

The subclinical impairments in attention and coordination seen in CHE also have significant impact on driving skills. Several studies have highlighted the effect CHE has on driving. Both on-road and simulator testing have consistently shown that driving performance is decreased in patients with CHE compared with patients with cirrhosis without CHE and healthy control subjects.[11–13] CHE patients were found to have a 22% chance of future traffic accidents compared with 3% in non-CHE patients with cirrhosis.[14]

Not all patients with CHE are affected. Up to 50% retain adequate driving capabilities and there is controversy on the value of routine psychometric testing to predict driving ability.[15] Several algorithms have been suggested to stratify driving risk; however, because of the lack of universally accepted testing the widespread application still remains difficult.[15] Standard therapies for CHE have been investigated and data support that driving ability can be improved with treatment.[16]

TREATMENT

Treatment of CHE is justified based on the impact of CHE on everyday life activities. In addition, once CHE develops 50% develop OHE within 3 years, which portends a graver prognosis.[17] After OHE develops cognitive impairment persists despite medical therapy or orthotopic liver transplantation.[18,19] Given the effects on well-being and outcomes, effective treatments strategies for CHE need to be developed. Several treatment algorithms have been proposed; however, exact timing and duration of therapy remains controversial because of the lack of standardized testing. Our group typically seeks out features of CHE from history, such as extreme fatigue, history of falls, accidents, difficulty maintaining employment, and if present empiric therapy is strongly considered. In the absence of these features we recommend psychometric testing for all patients with cirrhosis. **Fig. 1** shows a proposed algorithm for the detection and management of CHE.

Once CHE is diagnosed, there is no consensus as to the best therapeutic agent to use. Probiotics, nonabsorbable disaccharides, rifaximin, and L-ornithine L-asparatate (LOLA) have been the agents most studied to date. The data supporting the use of these agents are summarized in **Table 1**. The remainder of this article reviews the evidence to support specific agents in the treatment of CHE.

Probiotics

Ammonia production is often implicated in the development of HE. Probiotics help modulate ammonia production by decreasing urease activity of enteric bacteria and decreasing ammonia delivered to the portal venous system.[20] Probiotics decrease intestinal pH and improve gut nutrition causing favorable outcomes in ammonia modulation.[21] Several studies have investigated the use of probiotics in the treatment of CHE. A study by Liu and colleagues[22] compared fiber, fiber in combination with probiotics, and placebo. Psychometric test, stool pH, stool bacteriology, blood ammonia, and blood endotoxin levels were compared. When compared with placebo the combination of probiotics and fiber reversed 50% of CHE versus 13% with placebo. Statistically significant decreases in endogenous endotoxin and ammonia levels were seen in the treatment group. Of interest, Child-Pugh scores were found to have a statistically significant improvement in this small cohort (N = 20) in the combination group compared with placebo ($P = .04$).[22]

A study by Bajaj and colleagues[23] compared the effect of probiotics versus placebo on psychometric testing and QOL scores after 60 days of therapy. In the treatment arm of the study 70% of the patients showed reversal of CHE, whereas 0% of the patients in the placebo arm showed reversal ($P = .03$). In this study health-related QOL (HRQOL) was investigated using the Short Form 36. Probiotics were not found to impact HRQOL; however, some argue that if more sophisticated testing, such as

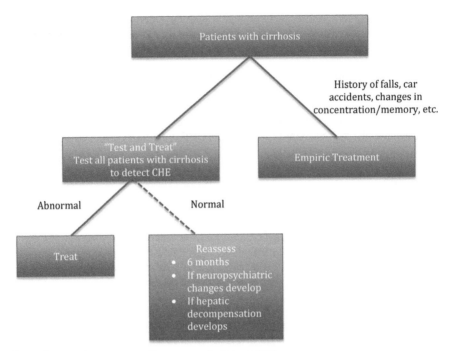

Fig. 1. Proposed strategy to diagnose and manage CHE.

the SIP, were used a different outcome may have been reached.[23] In the Bajaj and Liu studies, no patient in the active treatment group developed overt encephalopathy. In contrast, in the study by Bajaj, 25% of the placebo cohort developed OHE.[22,23]

To further support the use of probiotics, a recent prospective, randomized controlled study revealed that 50% fewer patients developed HE on probiotics compared with placebo.[24] A recent study by Vlachogiannakos and colleagues[25] presented in abstract form at the American Association for the Study of Liver Diseases meeting showed a 60% reduction in CHE in patients treated with *Lactobacillus plantarum* versus placebo. Meta-analysis has confirmed significant benefit of probiotics and a more favorable side effect profile compared with lactulose.[26] In addition to their excellent side effect profile, probiotics are also available commercially in yogurt without a prescription, giving them an advantage to other CHE therapies.[27] Given its favorable safety profile, accessibility, and beneficial effect on CHE reversal, probiotics are an attractive option for the management of CHE; however, the type and dose are unknown.

Lactulose

Nonabsorbable disaccharides have long been used in the treatment of OHE. Lactulose exerts multiple effects on ammonia metabolism including altering colonic pH affecting ammonia synthesis and absorption and glutamine uptake.[28] Several studies have investigated the impact of lactulose on the reversal of CHE. Dhiman and colleagues[29] used psychometric testing to compare lactulose with placebo. In their study, significant improvement was seen in psychometric testing with 57% of patients in the lactulose group showing resolution of CHE. A larger randomized

Table 1
Advantages and disadvantages of the therapeutic agents most studied for the management of covert hepatic encephalopathy

Drug	Advantages	Disadvantages	Evidence
Probiotics	Excellent tolerability Palatable food product Inexpensive No adverse events No prescription required Decreases CHE Prevents OHE	Multiple cultures Unregulated medical food Optimal dose and duration unknown	Liu et al[22] 50% vs 13% reversal of CHE (P<.05) Decreased ammonia and endotoxin levels (P = .05) Improved Child-Pugh scores (P = .04) Bajaj et al[23] 70% vs 0% with placebo in reversal of CHE (P = .03) 0% developed CHE vs 25% in placebo Lunia et al[24] 50% decrease in development of OHE (P<.05) Vlachogiannakos et al[25] 57% decrease in CHE vs placebo (P<.01) >80% compliance with therapy
Lactulose	Inexpensive Cost-effective Improves quality of life Decreases CHE	Diarrhea Abdominal pain Bloating Compliance (ADR) Poor palatability	Dhiman et al[29] 57% resolution of CHE Prasad et al[30] Improvement in psychometric testing (P = .04) HRQOL (Sickness Index Profile) improved (P = .002) Sharma and Sharma[31] 53% improved CHE during treatment
Rifaximin	Excellent tolerability Decreases CHE Improves quality of life	Expensive Not cost-effective	Bajaj et al[16] 91% vs 61% with placebo improved psychometric testing (P<.05) Psychosocial HRQOL improved (P = .04) Decreased driving errors on simulators (76% vs 31%; P = .13) Sidhu et al[35] 75% vs 20% placebo cleared CHE (P<.0001) Total HRQOL improved with 8 wk of therapy Bajaj et al[33] Not cost-effective at current pricing
LOLA, oral	Decreases rates of OHE 6 mo after discontinuation MELD/Child-Pugh scores improved 6 mo after discontinuation	Not shown to decrease CHE No improvement in QOL or depression/anxiety scores Limited experience	Alvares-da-Silva et al[37] No statistically significant change in CHE, QOL, or depression/anxiety scores OHE developed in 5% of LOLA vs 37.9% in placebo group 6 mo after discontinuation of therapy (P = .016) MELD/Child-Pugh scores improved 6 mo after discontinuation (P<.001)

Abbreviations: ADR, adverse drug reaction; HRQOL, health-related quality of life; MELD, Model for End-Stage Liver Disease.

controlled trial by Prasad and colleagues[30] also revealed a statistically significant impact on psychometric testing with the use of lactulose. HRQOL scores measured by SIP were also found to be significantly better in the group treated with lactulose. In this study, CHE negatively impacted 11 out of the 12 scales on the SIP and treatment with lactulose showed statistically significant improvement in the SIP in these domains. Further support for the prevalence of CHE in the population with cirrhosis was garnered in this study with 67.7% of Prasad and colleagues[30] outpatient population showing psychometric evidence of CHE. A recent study in patients with extrahepatic portal vein obstruction by Sharma and Sharma[31] confirmed the findings of the previous studies with over half of the patients treated with lactulose improving in psychometric studies.

Although effective, the study by Sharma and Sharma[31] also highlighted the substantial side effects of lactulose leading to a well-known dilemma in the use of lactulose (ie, is the benefit worth the cost). In Sharma's study, 30% of his cohort experienced gastrointestinal side effects including diarrhea, bloating, and taste alteration. Dose reduction was needed in four patients but no participant discontinued therapy during the study interval.[31] The findings of Prasad and colleagues[30] correlated with Sharma in that no serious adverse events were reported.[31] It is well established that the adverse events of lactulose are not trivial and have been shown to independently decrease QOL in patients undergoing treatment, which can affect long-term compliance.[32] Despite the side effect profile, lactulose has proved efficacy and is cost-effective in the treatment of CHE.[33]

Rifaximin

Rifaximin is a gut-specific, poorly absorbed antibiotic that has been used in a variety of gastrointestinal conditions from traveler's diarrhea to irritable bowel syndrome. Unlike traditional antimicrobial therapy, rifaximin is thought to modulate rather than eradicate bacteria. Complex studies of the metabolome of enteric bacteria during treatment with rifaximin show an alteration in bacterial function rather than number.[34]

Several studies have evaluated the efficacy of rifaximin in CHE. The 2011 study by Bajaj and colleagues[16] evaluated 41 patients randomized to rifaximin or placebo for 8 weeks. Rifaximin showed an improvement across a variety of study end points. Cognition improved in 91% of patients treated with rifaximin versus 61% in patients treated with placebo using a battery of neuropsychiatric tests. The psychosocial component of HRQOL was improved in patients treated with rifaximin.[16] This study also used driving simulators and found that rifaximin improved driving errors more effectively than placebo (76% vs 31%; $P = .13$).[16] There were no changes in ammonia levels between the groups but a clinically significant increase in the anti-inflammatory cytokine interleukin-10 was observed in the treatment group versus placebo, supporting the hypothesis of the mechanism of action of rifaximin in this study.[16]

A study performed by Sidhu and colleagues[35] with a slightly larger cohort (N = 94) treated patients with rifaximin and a significantly higher proportion (75% vs 20%) of patients in the treatment arm showed reversal of CHE on neuropsychiatric testing. A significant number of the five neuropsychiatric tests used in this study were improved within 2 weeks of therapeutic intervention. Similarly to the study by Bajaj, HRQOL was improved. After 8 weeks of therapy with rifaximin, HRQOL was improved as measured by total HRQOL scores.[35]

Rifaximin has excellent tolerability with few adverse events. In the study by Bajaj equal amounts of patients in the treatment and placebo arm experienced nausea, vomiting, and diarrhea, whereas more patients in the placebo arm developed headaches.[34] In the study by Sidhu and colleagues,[35] excellent tolerability was also shown. Only two patients in the treatment arm experienced adverse events. No patients in either study required dose reduction or treatment discontinuation because of rifaximin.[16,35] This tolerability represents a significant advantage over nonabsorbable disaccharides. The largest drawback to the routine use of rifaximin is cost. Investigators have looked at cost-effectiveness of rifaximin in comparison with other conventional treatments. Bajaj and colleagues[33] compared empiric treatment with various test-and-treat strategies and found that lactulose therapy was cost-effective across all testing variables. The use of the inhibitory control test to detect CHE and treatment with lactulose if testing was positive was the most cost-effective strategy. Rifaximin was not shown to be cost-effective at current prices.[33] Despite the cost constraints, rifaximin has excellent tolerability and efficacy in the treatment of CHE.

L-Ornithine-L-Aspartate

LOLA has been studied in oral and parenteral forms for the treatment of OHE with mixed results. LOLA is a peptide composed of ornithine and aspartate, two biologically active amino acids. These two amino acids enhance ammonia metabolism by activating enzymes in the urea cycle. It also acts as a substrate for glutamate synthesis to further detoxify ammonia.[36]

A recent study by Alvares-da-Silva and colleagues[37] evaluated 63 patients with CHE and randomized them in a double-blind fashion to oral LOLA versus placebo. Baseline evaluation included psychometric testing, critical flicker frequency, quantitative electroencephalogram, arterial ammonia, liver disease QOL assessment, and the Beck depression and anxiety surveys. After 60 days of treatment there was no improvement in patients receiving LOLA compared with the placebo arm. In contrast to studies using lactulose an overall increase in arterial ammonia concentration was seen in the placebo and LOLA groups. Similarly there was no statistically significant difference in QOL scores, anxiety, or depression scores.[37]

Although the results in reversal of CHE during active therapy were disappointing, a surprising finding was noted on follow-up. At 6 months after discontinuation of therapy, all study participants were evaluated to see if they had developed OHE. A statistically significant decrease was seen in the intervention group compared with placebo (5% vs 37.9%; $P = .016$).[37] In comparison with the placebo arm, the LOLA arm also had improvements in Child-Pugh and Model for End-Stage Liver Disease scores compared with the placebo arm. One theory behind the prevention of OHE is the ability of LOLA to modulate lipid and peptide metabolism. It is also theorized that ammonia metabolism is increased leading to increased glutamine production, which can stimulate hepatocyte growth factors.[36] More studies are needed to confirm these findings and to determine if longer treatment duration improves psychometric function and if improvements in liver function are sustained off therapy.

SUMMARY

Most patients with cirrhosis develop CHE over the course of their disease, resulting in significant decrement in QOL. Beneficial outcomes related to cognition, QOL, driving ability, and decrease in falls can be achieved if CHE is identified and treated. Despite its ubiquitous nature and significant potential for morbidity, the appropriate timing of diagnosis and treatment remains to be fully elucidated. Prophylactic therapy and test-and-treat options have been proposed but until standardized diagnostic tools exist to guide therapeutic decisions, CHE remains an underdiagnosed entity.

REFERENCES

1. Kappus MR, Bajaj JS. Covert hepatic encephalopathy: not as minimal as you might think. Clin Gastroenterol Hepatol 2012;10:1208–19.
2. Mullen KD, Prakash RV. Management of covert hepatic encephalopathy. Clin Liver Dis 2012;16:91–3.
3. Stinton LM, Jayakumar S. Minimal hepatic encephalopathy. Can J Gastroenterol 2013;27:572–4.
4. Bajaj JS, Etemadian A, Hafeezullah M, et al. Testing for minimal hepatic encephalopathy in the United States: an AASLD survey. Hepatology 2007;52:3259–65.
5. Arguedas MR, DeLawrence TG, McGuire BM. Influence of hepatic encephalopathy on health-related quality of life in patients with cirrhosis. Dig Dis Sci 2003; 48:1622–6.
6. Groeneweg M, Quero JC, Bruijn I, et al. Subclinical hepatic encephalopathy impairs daily functioning. Hepatology 1998;28:45–9.
7. Peeters G, Van Schoo NM, Lips P. Fall risk: the clinical relevance of falls and how to integrate fall risk with fracture risk. Best Pract Res Clin Rheumatol 2009;23: 797–804.
8. Weisenborn K, Ennen JC, Schomerus H, et al. Neuropsychological characterization of hepatic encephalopathy. J Hepatol 2001;34:768–73.
9. Román E, Córdoba J, Torrens M, et al. Minimal hepatic encephalopathy is associated with falls. Am J Gastroenterol 2011;106:476–82.
10. Schomerus H, Hamster W. Quality of life in cirrhotics with minimal hepatic encephalopathy. Metab Brain Dis 2001;16:37–41.
11. Wein C, Koch H, Popp B, et al. Minimal hepatic encephalopathy impairs fitness to drive. Hepatology 2004;39:739–45.
12. Bajaj JS, Hafeezullah M, Hoffman RG, et al. Minimal hepatic encephalopathy: a vehicle for accidents and traffic violations. Am J Gastroenterol 2007;102:1903–9.
13. Kim Y, Park G, Lee M, et al. Impairment of driving ability and neuropsychological function in patients with MHE disease. Cyberpsychol Behav 2009;12:433–6.
14. Bajaj JS, Saeian K, Schubert CM, et al. Minimal hepatic encephalopathy is associated with motor vehicle crashes: the reality beyond the driving test. Hepatology 2009;50:1175–83.
15. Prakash RV, Brown TA, Mullen KD. Minimal hepatic encephalopathy and driving: is the genie out of the bottle. Am J Gastroenterol 2011;106:1415–6.
16. Bajaj JS, Heuman DM, Wade JB, et al. Rifaximin improves driving simulator performance in a randomized trial of patients with minimal hepatic encephalopathy. Gastroenterology 2011;140:478–87.
17. Hartman IJ, Groeneweg M, Quero JC, et al. The prognostic significance of subclinical hepatic encephalopathy. Am J Gastroenterol 2000;95:2029–34.
18. Bajaj JS, Schubert CM, Heuman DM, et al. Persistence of cognitive impairment after resolution of overt hepatic encephalopathy. Gastroenterology 2010;138: 2332–40.
19. Garcia-Martinez R, ROvira A, Alonso J, et al. Hepatic encephalopathy is associated with posttransplant cognitive function and brain volume. Liver Transpl 2011; 17:38–46.
20. Prakash RK, Kanna S, Mullen K. Evolving concepts: the negative effect of minimal hepatic encephalopathy and role for prophylaxis in patients with cirrhosis. Clin Ther 2013;35:1458–73.
21. Toapanta-Yanchapaxi L, López-Velázquez JA, Uribe M, et al. Minimal hepatic encephalopathy. Should we treat it? Ann Hepatol 2013;12:487–92.

22. Liu Q, Duan ZP, Ha DK, et al. Symbiotic modulation of gut flora: effect on minimal hepatic encephalopathy in patients with cirrhosis. Hepatology 2004;39:1441–9.
23. Bajaj JS, Saeian K, Christensen KM, et al. Probiotic yogurt for the treatment of minimal hepatic encephalopathy. Am J Gastroenterol 2008;103:1707–15.
24. Lunia MK, Sharma BC, Sharma P, et al. Probiotics prevent hepatic encephalopathy in patients with cirrhosis: a randomized controlled trial. Clin Gastroenterol Hepatol 2014;12:1003–8.
25. Vlachogiannakos J, Vasianopoulou P, Viazis N, et al. The role of probiotics in the treatment of minimal hepatic encephalopathy. A prospective, randomized placebo-controlled, double-blind study. Hepatology 2014;60:376A.
26. Shukla S, Shukla A, Mehboob S, et al. Meta-analysis: the effects of gut flora modulation using prebiotics, probiotics and xenobiotics on minimal hepatic encephalopathy. Aliment Pharmacol Ther 2011;33:662–71.
27. Alfawaz HA, Aljumah AA. What improves minimal hepatic encephalopathy: probiotic yogurt, protein restriction or nonabsorbable disaccharides? Saudi J Gastroenterol 2012;18:153–4.
28. Zhan T, Stremmel W. The diagnosis and treatment of minimal hepatic encephalopathy. Dtsch Arztebl Int 2012;109:180–7.
29. Dhiman RK, Sawhney MS, Chaula YK, et al. Efficacy of lactulose in cirrhotic patients with subclinical hepatic encephalopathy. Dig Dis Sci 2000;45:1549–52.
30. Prasad S, Dhiman R, Duseja A, et al. Lactulose improves cognitive functions and health-related quality of life in patients with cirrhosis who have minimal hepatic encephalopathy. Hepatology 2007;45:549–59.
31. Sharma P, Sharma BC. Lactulose for minimal hepatic encephalopathy in patients with extrahepatic portal vein obstruction. Saudi J Gastroenterol 2012;18:168–72.
32. Kalaitzakis E, SImren M, Olsson R, et al. Gastrointestinal symptoms in patients with liver cirrhosis: associations with nutritional status and health related quality of life. Scand J Gastroenterol 2006;41:1464–72.
33. Bajaj JS, Pinkerton SD, Sanyal AJ, et al. Diagnosis and treatment of minimal hepatic encephalopathy to prevent motor vehicle accidents: a cost-effectiveness analysis. Hepatology 2012;55:1164–71.
34. Bajaj JS, Heuman DM, Sanyal AJ, et al. Modulation of the metabiome by rifaximin in patients with cirrhosis and minimal hepatic encephalopathy. PLoS One 2013;8:e60042.
35. Sidhu SS, Goyal O, Mishra BP, et al. Rifaximin improves psychometric performance and health-related quality of life in patients with minimal hepatic encephalopathy (the RIME Trial). Am J Gastroenterol 2011;106:307–16.
36. Tomiya T. Treatment for minimal hepatic encephalopathy: are we ghost busters. Hepatol Res 2014;44:937–9.
37. Alvares-da-Silva MR, Araujo A, Vicenzi JR, et al. Oral L-ornithine-L-aspartate in minimal hepatic encephalopathy: a randomized, double-blind, placebo-controlled trial. Hepatol Res 2014;44:956–63.

Diets in Encephalopathy

George G. Abdelsayed, MD

KEYWORDS

- Diet • Encephalopathy • End-stage liver disease • Malnutrition

KEY POINTS

- As many as 80% of patients with end-stage liver disease and hepatic encephalopathy have significant protein-calorie malnutrition.
- Because of the severe hypercatabolic state of cirrhosis, the provision of liberal amounts of carbohydrate (at least 35 to 40 kcal/kg per day), and between 1.2 and 1.6 g/kg of protein is necessary.
- Protein restriction is not recommended; branched-chain amino acid supplementation and vegetable protein are associated with improved outcomes.
- Dietary supplementation with vitamins, minerals (with the notable exception of zinc) and probiotics should be decided on a case-by-case basis.

INTRODUCTION

Hepatic encephalopathy (HE) is a disorder of reversible impairment of cerebral function in patients with acute or chronic hepatic failure or when the portal circulation is bypassed by the creation of portosystemic shunts. The disorder carries a dismal prognosis with a 40% survival at 1 year.[1] Up to 80% of patients with cirrhosis may have clinically undetectable or minimal HE. This article discusses current concepts in the dietary and nutritional management of HE.

GENERAL

In order to understand the rationale behind dietary management in HE, it is important to briefly review the pathophysiology of HE. The liver plays a central role in the detoxification and neutralization of many toxic substances absorbed from the gastrointestinal tract, as well as other substances produced as byproducts of normal daily metabolism. The toxins enter the portal circulation through the low-flow hepatic sinusoids. The detoxification process occurs in the hepatocytes. Among the central toxins studied is ammonia. Ammonia is absorbed by both neurons and astrocytes. The astrocytes convert the ammonia to glutamine to minimize its toxic effects on the neurons. Ammonia is toxic to both astrocytes and neurons. It is the astrocyte (the glial cells of the central nervous system) that is pivotal in providing adequate nutrition to

Disclosure: The author has nothing to disclose.
475 Seaview Avenue, Staten Island, NY 10305, USA
E-mail address: g-abd@hotmail.com

Clin Liver Dis 19 (2015) 497–505
http://dx.doi.org/10.1016/j.cld.2015.05.001
liver.theclinics.com
1089-3261/15/$ – see front matter © 2015 Elsevier Inc. All rights reserved.

neurons.[2] **Fig. 1** shows the metabolism of ammonia and its role in HE and inflammation. Although the exact mechanisms of damage to neurons and astrocytes by toxins, including ammonia, in HE is not understood, it is known that astrocyte swelling with resultant cerebral edema is key in the pathophysiology of HE associated with acute liver failure.[3]

As many as 80% of patients with end-stage liver disease have varying degrees of protein-calorie malnutrition, caused by multiple factors (**Fig. 2**).[4] This degree of protein-calorie malnutrition may be as high as 25% in patients who are Child-Pugh class A.[5] Because of significant fluid retention, hypoalbuminemia, and loss of muscle mass, it is not always possible to use objective parameters to assess the degree of malnutrition in decompensated cirrhotic patients. In 2006, The European Society for Clinical Nutrition and Metabolism published guidelines on nutrition support for patients with liver disease for inpatients and outpatients.[6] Because of the aforementioned difficulties of applying objective parameters, simple bedside methods such as subjective global assessment or anthropometry are used to identify high-risk patients.[7] Wherever possible, enteral nutrition is strongly favored rather than parenteral nutrition. Parenteral nutrition may be indicated in situations of ongoing sepsis, complete bowel obstruction or persistent vomiting, diarrhea, or aspiration. Wherever possible, the benefits of parenteral nutrition must be carefully weighed against the risks, particularly septic and fluid overload complications.[8]

CARBOHYDRATE INTAKE

Because of the severe anorexia of cirrhosis, many patients inadvertently follow a hypocaloric diet. Among the contributing factors are the circulation of anorexigenic proinflammatory intermediaries, such as the interleukins and tumor necrosis factor alpha, and impaired gastric distensibility from ascites. With a resting energy expenditure 120% above baseline, and the hypermetabolic/catabolic state of cirrhosis, carbohydrate intake must necessarily be liberalized. Patients with cirrhosis are also glycogen depleted. The hyperglucagonemia and insulin resistance in these patients impairs glycogenolysis, which is combined with the already depleted glycogen stores in the liver. Gluconeogenesis therefore becomes the preferred method for the replenishment of glucose. This process consequently results in a severe depletion of amino acid stores in the liver and skeletal muscle. Although this may occur in healthy

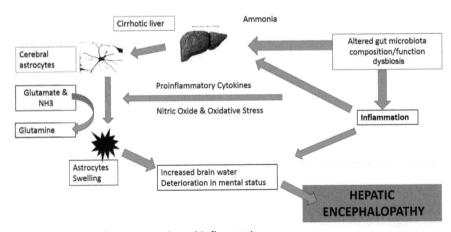

Fig. 1. Pathophysiology: ammonia and inflammation.

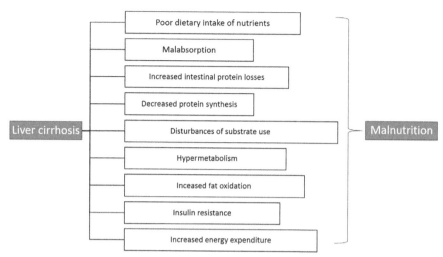

Fig. 2. Factors contributing to malnutrition in end-stage liver failure.

individuals following a prolonged fast (>3 days), in a cirrhotic patient this can occur following an overnight fast.[9,10] With this in mind, the ultimate goal is to slow down the catabolic process and to achieve a state of anabolism. At a minimum, to achieve anabolism, or at least to avoid catabolism, energy requirements should consist of 35 to 40 kcal/kg/d. Protein intake (discussed later) should be 1.2 to 1.6 g/kg/d or 350 to 480 kcal of the total. Because of the need to provide a continuous flow of nutrients for these patients, 3 meals per day are not adequate. Instead, 4 to 6 meals, including snacks with foods rich in carbohydrates, is preferred.[11] Because diets low in sodium tend to be calorie restricted, a diet providing the equivalent of 2 g of sodium is prudent to ensure adequate compliance with a hypercaloric diet.

Restriction of carbohydrate intake in patients with end-stage liver disease and HE is generally not prudent, even in patients with diabetes mellitus (probably 40%–50% of all patients with end-stage liver disease). In cirrhotic diabetics, hyperinsulinemia and insulin resistance are exacerbated. Although the hyperinsulinemia may cause a tendency to promote hypoglycemia, especially in alcoholics who may have an inhibition of gluconeogenesis, this generally does not commonly occur because of insulin resistance.[12,13]

PROTEIN INTAKE: NORMAL OR RESTRICTED?

With their reduced muscle mass, severe anorexia, nausea, reduced oral intake, malabsorption, and the inherent hypermetabolic/catabolic state, patients with advanced and/ or decompensated liver disease are severely malnourished and protein depleted. Despite this, protein restriction (generally defined as a daily protein intake of 20 g) has historically been advocated for these patients. The older practice advocated a gradual increase in protein intake to a limit of 0.8 to 1.0 g/kg of body weight in an effort to achieve positive nitrogen balance.[14] This approach is flawed because, even in patients with stable cirrhosis, the protein requirements are higher than normal: about 1.2 g/kg dry bodyweight and even higher in more advanced malnutrition.[15] Low-protein diets tend to exacerbate preexisting protein-calorie malnutrition, and lead to worse outcomes. Protein restriction may be considered in some patients immediately following a severe episode of acute encephalopathy, such as in acute hepatic failure, and even then only for a short initial period. Because malnutrition, especially protein-calorie malnutrition, is common in liver disease, protein restriction is rarely justified.

AROMATIC AND BRANCHED-CHAIN AMINO ACIDS: VEGETABLE VERSUS ANIMAL PROTEIN

As mentioned previously, between 60% and 90% of patients with advanced cirrhosis present with protein-energy malnutrition, manifested by cachexia, low serum albumin level, and low muscle mass. This state of protein-energy malnutrition is worsened by the anorexia of cirrhosis. Ultimately these patients become hyperglucagonemic. Persistent hyperglucagonemia results in a worsening of catabolic activity, eventually aggravating the anorexia/cachexia vicious cycle.[16] Because these patients are less able to metabolize glucose efficiently, they rely more heavily on the use of branched-chain amino acids (BCAAs), which include leucine, isoleucine, and valine, as an efficient energy source. BCAAs quickly become depleted from the circulation, as they are taken up by the starving skeletal muscle, which uses them for the resynthesis of glutamine. Glutamine in turn is essential for the clearance of ammonia, which is not cleared efficiently by the failing liver.[17] Furthermore, patients with advanced cirrhosis are unable to use the aromatic amino acids (tyrosine, tryptophan, and phenylalanine), which leads to an increase in the aromatic amino acids relative to the BCAAs.[18(p484)] This unfavorable ratio allows more aromatic amino acids to enter the blood-brain barrier, where they act as substrates for the production of false neurotransmitters, such as octopamine, tyramine, and phenylethanolamine. Serotonin (a true neurotransmitter) production may also increase. These neurotransmitters contribute to the production of more ammonia. BCAA supplementation is thought to facilitate ammonia detoxification by supporting the increased synthesis of glutamine, which is a non–branched-chain amino acid, in skeletal muscle. This process also results in diminishing the influx of the aromatic amino acids across the blood-brain barrier.[18(p485)]

Another major advantage of BCAA supplementation is the amelioration of malnutrition in cirrhosis. BCAA supplementation can reduce protein loss, and support can increase protein synthesis.[19] Leucine seems to be the most efficient, by stimulating multiple pathways of protein synthesis.[18(pp486,487)] Insulin deficiency and insulin resistance are common in advanced cirrhosis, insulin resistance being primarily related to hyperglucagonemia. BCAA supplementation ameliorates the hyperglucagonemic state by stimulating insulin released by the pancreatic beta cells and increasing insulin sensitivity. It has been shown in some animal models that this is accomplished by induction of transcription of the glucose transporter type 2 (GLUT2) transporter and liver-type glucokinase.[18] Therefore, BCAA supplementation seems to inhibit protein breakdown, improve use of glucose, and stimulate protein synthesis. These effects help to downregulate gluconeogenesis. This downregulation process is particularly important in the kidney, where up to 28% of glucose is released into the bloodstream.[20]

Patients with cirrhosis also have impaired immune defense mechanisms, which are characterized primarily by decreased intracellular killing and impaired phagocytic activity. BCAA supplementation may enhance liver cell regeneration by secretion of growth factors from stellate cells.[19] BCAA supplementation may also promote albumin synthesis as well as protein and glycogen synthesis by skeletal muscle. Marchesini and colleagues[21(p1600)] showed an improvement in certain parameters, such as an increase in serum albumin and a decrease in the serum bilirubin, with BCAA supplementation.

Although the utility of BCAAs has been debated for many years, several large-scale studies have shown that long-term, oral BCAA supplementation improves survival in patients with end-stage liver disease and HE by decreasing certain fatal outcomes, such as gastrointestinal bleeding and hepatic failure.[22] A multicenter, randomized, double-blind controlled trial compared patients with advanced cirrhosis taking BCAAs versus controls (a milk protein composed of maltodextrins and lactalbumin) for amelioration of liver failure and survival in patients on BCAAs ($P = .039$).[21(p1598)] A worsening of encephalopathy was also seen in half of the patients in the casein group but in only 1 patient in the BCAA group.[23] Studies have also shown a decrease in hospital admission rates, improvement in liver function tests, and lower infection rates with BCAA supplementation.[24]

BCAAs make up approximately 25% of the protein content of most foods in the United States. The highest content is seen in casein whey protein of dairy products and vegetables such as corn and mushrooms. Other sources high in BCAAs include peanuts, egg albumin, and brown rice.[21(p1597)] Oral supplementation of BCAAs, although beneficial, tends to be unpalatable and requires patients to drink large volumes of water, which may not be desirable in patients with decompensated cirrhosis. The principal downside of BCAA supplementation is their high cost.[25] Bloating, abdominal distention, diarrhea, and vomiting are seen in up to 15% of patients. Although self-limiting, they can be ameliorated and palatability improved if they are supplemented by way of dairy products, eggs, or vegetables.[21(p1600)] Late-night administration of BCAAs seems to confer a benefit.[26]

The source of protein (meat vs vegetable) has been studied by several investigators. Meat-derived protein contains a significantly higher amount of the amino acid methionine, a sulfur-containing amino acid. Methionine is metabolized by gut bacteria to products referred to as mercaptans, which are precursors of the false neurotransmitters mentioned previously. Vegetable-derived proteins have a higher content of BCAAs and significantly lower quantities of methionine, and are therefore better tolerated in patients with cirrhosis and HE. It has been shown that cirrhotic patients who consume higher quantities of vegetable versus meat protein have an overall clinical improvement, decreased HE index scores, improved performance on intellectual tasks, and decreased ammonia levels. This improvement was further enhanced with optimal use of lactulose.[27,28]

Other studies have suggested that BCAAs may favorably affect intestinal transit, decrease gastric transit time, and increase intraluminal gut pH.[29] A recommended daily intake of 30 to 40 g of vegetable protein has been found to be effective in most patients with end-stage liver disease and HE.[28]

FAT, VITAMINS, SUPPLEMENTS, PROBIOTICS, FIBER

There is evidence of increased fat absorption in patients with end-stage liver disease. Fat is absorbed primarily through the portal venous system. This increased absorption, coupled with the impairment in hepatic very-low-density lipoprotein release, contributes to the increased hepatic fat storage.[30] It is prudent to keep fat intake at less than 30% of the total calories, with less than 10% of the total as saturated fat. A diet rich in fiber is also recommended, because cirrhotic patients are more prone to constipation.

Vitamin supplementation in patients with cirrhosis and end-stage liver disease should be individualized.[12] For example, osteoporosis is common in patients with end-stage liver disease, particularly in patients with risk factors such as cigarette smoking and older age. Calcium should be supplemented at a dose of 1200 to 1500 mg and 400 to 800 IU of vitamin D should be given, especially in patients with cholestasis. In patients with established osteoporosis, the addition of bisphosphonates may also be advised. Vitamin A in a dose of 100,000 to 200,000 IU may be prescribed for patients with symptoms of night blindness.[12]

Table 1		
Metabolic alterations leading to malnutrition in end-stage liver failure		
Protein	**Carbohydrate**	**Fat**
Increased use of BCAAs	Decreased hepatic and skeletal	Increased lipolysis
Decreased ureagenesis	muscle glycogen synthesis	Increased ketogenesis
Increased catabolism	Glucose intolerance and insulin	Enhanced turnover and
	resistance	oxidation of fatty acids
	Increased gluconeogenesis	

Zinc was most recently studied by Takoma and colleagues[31] in 2010. Most patients with cirrhosis are deficient in zinc, and this is particularly problematic in alcoholic patients. Takoma and colleagues[31] randomized patients with cirrhosis and HE grades I and II who were refractory to standard treatment to receive zinc in addition to lactulose and BCAAs versus no zinc with lactulose and BCAAs. Patients were followed for 6 months to determine the effect on quality of life and HE. HE improved in 54% of patients compared with 26% of patients in the zinc versus No-zinc arms, with 16 zinc-treated patients improving to achieve an encephalopathy grade of zero. Coadministration of BCAAs with carnitine and zinc was also shown by Holececk[18] to increase ammonia metabolism and clearance, further reducing encephalopathy symptoms.[31]

Probiotics are live microbiota with beneficial effects to the host. Prebiotics are substances that promote the growth of beneficial bacteria within the intestinal microbiome. Their benefits include denying harmful bacteria needed metabolic substrates, and the provision of necessary fermentation products to beneficial bacteria. The ultimate desired result is an increase in the intestinal flora of lactic acid–type bacteria at the expense of harmful flora. Several investigators have examined the concept of treating HE with probiotics.[32,33] Subsequently, such benefits have been shown by various investigators. Bajaj and colleagues[34] showed some reversal of minimal HE with probiotics. A significant reduction of blood ammonia level was shown by other investigators.[35] Use of probiotics was also shown to have beneficial effects on synthetic markers, including the serum bilirubin, albumin, and prothrombin time.[35] One study showed improved hepatic synthetic function and serum transaminase levels in patients with hepatitis C and alcohol-related cirrhosis.[36] Given their demonstrated efficacy and acceptable tolerability, they are increasingly used in the management of HE. **Table 1** summarizes metabolic alterations leading to malnutrition in end-stage liver failure, and **Table 2** summarizes nutritional recommendations for the management of HE in the end-stage liver.

Table 2	
Nutritional recommendations for the management of HE in end-stage liver failure	
Substrate	**Recommendation**
Protein	1.2–1.5 g/kg body weight/d[a]
Energy	35–40 kcal/kg/d
BCAA	In severely protein-intolerant patients
Antioxidant and vitamin	Multivitamin supplements
Probiotics, prebiotics	Increasing use for ammonia level–lowering and antiinflammatory actions

[a] In severely protein-intolerant patients, protein may be reduced for short periods of time, particularly in grade III to IV HE.

SUMMARY

HE is a serious complication of decompensated end-stage liver disease. Patients with HE have serious nutritional problems, with at least 80% having varying degrees of protein-calorie malnutrition. The hypercatabolism and increased energy expenditure in these patients coupled with hyperglucagonemia and insulin resistance poses important nutritional challenges. A liberal caloric intake, with 2500 to 3000 kcal per day, and a protein intake of 1.2 to 1.6 g/kg per day are recommended. Protein restriction (defined as 20 g or less of protein intake per day) should be discouraged, except in the initial management of severe acute HE. Because of the low ratio of BCAAs to aromatic amino acids in these patients, BCAA supplementation is recommended. Proteins from a vegetable source confer the greatest benefit relative to proteins from an animal source, partly because of the higher content of BCAAs and lower content of methionine in vegetable protein. Supplementation of vitamins, particularly the fat-soluble vitamins A and D, should be considered on a case-by-case basis. Zinc supplementation, with BCAAs and consistent use of lactulose, as well as probiotics has also been shown to be beneficial.

REFERENCES

1. Bustamante J, Rimola A, Ventura PJ, et al. Prognostic significance of hepatic encephalopathy in patients with cirrhosis. J Hepatol 1999;30:890–5.
2. Reddy PV, Rama Rao KV, Norenberg MD. J Neurosci Res 2009;87:2677–85.
3. Cordoba J, Minguez B. hepatic encephalopathy. Semin Liver Dis 2008;28:70–80.
4. Kalaitzakis E, Simren M, Olsson R, et al. Gastrointestinal symptoms in patients with liver cirrhosis: associations with nutritional status and health-related quality-of-life. Can J Gastroenterol 2006;41:1464–72.
5. Guglielmi FW, Panella C, Buda A, et al. Nutritional state and energy balance in cirrhotic take patients with or without hypermetabolism. Multicentre perspective study by the 'Nutritional Problems in Gastroenterology' section of the Italian Society of Gastroenterology (SIGE). Dig Liver Dis 2005;37:681–8.
6. Figueiredo FA, De Mello Perez R, Kondo M. Effect of liver cirrhosis on body composition: evidence of significant depletion even in mild disease. J Gastroenterol Hepatol 2005;105:1839–45.
7. Plauth M, Cabre E, Riggio O, et al. ESPEN guidelines on enteral nutrition: liver disease. Clin Nutr 2006;25:285–94.
8. Cabre E, Gassull MA. Nutrition in liver disease. Curr Opin Clin Nutr Metab Care 2005;8:545–51.
9. Owen OE, Reiche FA, Mozzoli MA, et al. Hepatic, gut and renal substrate flux rates in patients with hepatic cirrhosis. J Clin Invest 1981;68:240–52.
10. Owen OE, Trapp VE, Reichard GA Jr, et al. Nature and quantity of fuels consumed in patients with alcoholic cirrhosis. J Clin Invest 1983;72:1821–32.
11. Nakaya Y, Okita K, Suzuki K, et al. BCAA-enriched snack improves nutritional state of cirrhosis. Nutrition 2007;23:113–20.
12. Gundling F, Teich N, Strebel HM, et al. Ernahrung bei leberzirrhose. Med Klin 2007;102:435–44.
13. Swart GR, Zillikens MC, van Vuure JK, et al. Effect of a late evening meal on nitrogen balance in patients with cirrhosis of the liver. BMJ 1989;299:1202–3.
14. Andres T. Hepatic encephalopathy. In: Bircher J, Benhamou P, McIntyre N, et al, editors. Oxford textbook of clinical hepatology. 2nd edition. Oxford (United Kingdom): Oxford University Press; 1999. p. 765–83.

15. Plauth M, Merli M, Kondrup J, et al. ESPEN guidelines for nutrition in disease and transplantation. Clin Nutr 1997;16:43–55.

16. Bianchi G, Marzocchi R, Agostini F, et al. Update on branched-chain amino acid supplementation in liver diseases. Curr Opin Gastroenterol 2005;21:197. Available at: http://journals.lww.com/co-gastroenterology/Abstract/2005/03000/Update_on_branched_chain_amino_acid.12.aspx.

17. Moriwaki H, Miwa Y, Tajika M, et al. Branched-chain amino acids as a protein- and energy-source in liver cirrhosis. Biochem Biophys Res Commun 2004;313:405–7.

18. Holececk M. Three targets of branched chain amino acid supplementation in the treatment of liver disease. Nutrition 2010;26:484–90.

19. Higuchi N, Kato M, Masayuki M, et al. Potential role of branched chain amino acids in glucose metabolism through the accelerated induction of the glucose-sensing apparatus in the liver. J Cell Biochem 2010;112(1):30–8.

20. Gonzelez RR, Zweig S, Rao J, et al. Octreotide therapy for recurrent refractory hypoglycemia due to sulfonylurea in diabetes-related kidney failure. Endocr Pract 2007;13(4):1–7.

21. Marchesini G, Marzocchi R, Noia M, et al. Branched-chain amino acid supplementation in liver diseases. J Nutr 2005;135(Suppl 6):1569S–601S.

22. Yoshida T, Muto Y, Moriwaki H, et al. Effect of long-term oral supplementation with branched-chain amino acid granules on the prognosis of liver cirrhosis. Gastroenterol Jpn 1989;24:692–8.

23. Bianchi G, Marzocchi R, Agostini F, et al. Update on nutritional supplementation with branched-chain amino acids. Curr Opin Clin Nutr Metab Care 2005;8:83–7.

24. Charlton M. branched-chain amino acid enriched supplements as therapy for liver disease. J Nutr 2006;136(Suppl):295S–8S.

25. Eriksson LS, Persson A, Wahren J. Branched-chain amino acids in the treatment of chronic hepatic encephalopathy. Gut 1982;23(10):801–6.

26. Yamauchi M, Takeda K, Sakamoto K, et al. Effect of oral branched chain amino acid supplementation in the late evening on the nutritional state of patients with liver cirrhosis. Hepatol Res 2001;21:199–204.

27. Greenberger NJ, Carley J, Schenker S, et al. Effect of vegetable and animal protein diets in chronic hepatic encephalopathy. Am J Dig Dis 1977;32(10):845–55.

28. Bianchi GP, Marchesini G, Fabbri A, et al. Vegetable versus animal protein diet in cirrhotic patients with chronic encephalopathy. A randomized cross-over comparison. J Intern Med 1933;233(5):385–92.

29. Keshavarzian A, Meek J, Sutton C, et al. Dietary protein supplementation from vegetable sources in the management of chronic portal systemic encephalopathy. Am J Gastroenterol 1984;79(12):945–9.

30. Cabré E, Hernández-Pérez JM, Fluvià L, et al. Absorption and transport of dietary long-chain fatty acids in cirrhosis: a stable isotope tracing study. Am J Clin Nutr 2005;81:692–701.

31. Takoma Y, Nouso K, Makino Y, et al. Clinical trial: oral zinc in hepatic encephalopathy. Aliment Pharmacol Ther 2010;32:1080–90.

32. Macbeth WA, Kass EN, Mcdermott WV. Treatment of hepatic encephalopathy by alteration of intestinal flora with *Lactobacillus acidophilus*. Lancet 1965; 285(7382):399–403.

33. Loguercio C, Abbiati R, Rinaldi M, et al. Long-term effects of *Enterococcus faecium* SF68 versus lactulose in the treatment of patients with cirrhosis and grade 1-2 hepatic encephalopathy. J Hepatol 1995;23(1):39.

34. Bajaj JS, Saeian K, Christensen KM, et al. Probiotic yogurt for the treatment of minimal hepatic encephalopathy. Am J Gastroenterol 2008;103:1707–15.

35. Liu Q, Duan ZP, Ha DK, et al. Synbiotic modulation of gut flora: effect on minimal hepatic encephalopathy in patients with cirrhosis. Hepatology 2004;39(5): 1441–9.
36. Loguercio C, Federico A, Tuccillo C, et al. Beneficial effects of a probiotic VSL3 on parameters of liver dysfunction in chronic liver diseases. J Clin Gastroenterol 2005;39:540–3.

The Role of Sarcopenia and Frailty in Hepatic Encephalopathy Management

Catherine Lucero, MD, Elizabeth C. Verna, MD, MS*

KEYWORDS

- Frailty • Sarcopenia • Hepatic encephalopathy

KEY POINTS

- There are now several metrics that can be used to evaluate and quantify frailty and sarcopenia, although currently there is no validated disease-specific model for patients with cirrhosis.
- Frailty and sarcopenia may lead to an increased risk of hyperammonemia and clinically apparent hepatic encephalopathy, as well as pretransplant and posttransplant mortality.
- There is an important pathophysiologic relationship between hepatic encephalopathy and abnormalities in nutritional status and muscle metabolism in patients with cirrhosis, which could be targeted for therapeutic intervention.

INTRODUCTION

Cirrhosis is a chronic, debilitating disease that in its advanced stages, results in depletion of muscle mass, loss of functional status, susceptibility to severe infection, and complications that may ultimately be life-threatening. The concepts of frailty and sarcopenia have only recently been quantitatively applied to patients with cirrhosis, and there are currently no validated disease-specific measures for sarcopenia in patients with cirrhosis. However, when quantitative measures, including combinations of biochemical, radiographic, and physical performance measures, have been studied, there is now evidence that these syndromes affect a significant proportion of patients with cirrhosis and negatively impact patient outcomes.[1–6]

As described in detail in this issue of *Clinics in Liver Disease*, hepatic encephalopathy (HE) entails a spectrum of neuropsychiatric abnormalities seen in patients with

The authors have nothing to disclose.
Division of Digestive and Liver Diseases, Department of Medicine, Center for Liver Disease and Transplantation, Columbia University College of Physicians and Surgeons, 622 West 168th Street, PH 14-105, New York, NY 10032, USA
* Corresponding author.
E-mail address: ev77@columbia.edu

liver dysfunction and/or portosystemic shunting and in its most subtle form, termed "minimal" HE, may affect up to 80% of patients with cirrhosis.[7] Although the complex pathogenesis of HE is reviewed elsewhere in this issue, because of the significant involvement of skeletal muscle in ammonia metabolism[8] and the potential for increased glutamine and therefore ammonia load in the setting of muscle protein catabolism,[9] there is growing interest in the role of sarcopenia in the pathogenesis of HE, which may represent a target for therapeutic interventions.

DEFINING AND MEASURING FRAILTY AND SARCOPENIA

Sarcopenia is defined as the loss of skeletal muscle mass, quality, and strength normally associated with aging but also often present in the setting of debilitating chronic illness, such as cirrhosis.[10,11] Sarcopenia is a key component of *frailty*, the biologic syndrome of decreased reserve and resistance to stressors, resulting from cumulative declines across multiple physiologic systems, leading to vulnerability to adverse outcomes.[12] There are significant limitations in the diagnosis of sarcopenia and frailty in patients with cirrhosis because of the lack of objectivity and reproducibility of available tests. This is especially true for functional testing, which likely best links these concepts to relevant disease phenotypes. Although patients with cirrhosis often have changes in body composition, including decreased muscle and adipose tissue mass, extracellular fluid volume expansion and baseline obesity can mask the conventional physical findings in patients with sarcopenia. Physical examination may lack sensitivity in the presence of ascites, which impacts the calculation of the body mass index (BMI) and could lead to misrepresentation of nutritional status. Laboratory tests, including albumin, pre-albumin, and prothrombin time, may overestimate the prevalence of malnutrition due to the synthetic dysfunction seen in cirrhosis. In addition, concurrent HE may significantly limit the ability of individual patients to answer questions and perform physical tests. Despite these limitations, there is a growing literature using a variety of techniques to quantify frailty and sarcopenia in patients with cirrhosis.

Sarcopenia

The European Working Group on Sarcopenia consensus statement defines sarcopenia as a syndrome characterized by progressive and generalized loss of skeletal muscle mass and strength that can lead to adverse outcomes, such as physical disability, poor quality of life, and death.[11] The diagnosis requires documentation of both low muscle mass and function, although radiographic assessment of muscle mass is often used, and similar concepts have previously been referred to as states such as "protein-calorie malnutrition."[13–15] Although the diagnostic criteria reported varies, sarcopenia is often defined as muscle mass two standard deviations below sex-specific means of healthy adults,[11] with loss of up to 20% to 60% of skeletal muscle mass and strength.[9,14,16]

Despite this definition, most studies of sarcopenia in patients with cirrhosis focus on objective measures of muscle mass alone (**Table 1**). Several approaches to measurement of muscle mass have been studied, the most commonly used being cross-sectional measurement of muscle areas, such as the psoas muscle area or the skeletal muscle index, calculated from radiographic images at a uniform vertebral level (such as L3 or L4 spine, **Fig. 1**).[2,5,10,17,18] In addition, several techniques that attempt to indirectly quantify measure of body composition also have been used. Bioimpedance analysis,[11,19] which incorporates analysis of total body water as well as muscle and fat mass, has been used though the accuracy of this test may be impaired by the marked extracellular volume expansion in many patients with cirrhosis. In addition,

Table 1
Measures of sarcopenia and frailty

Syndrome	Disease Measure	Components	Abnormal Test Result Range	Considerations for Patients with Cirrhosis	Examples in the Literature
Sarcopenia	Psoas muscle area/Skeletal muscle index	Cross-sectional imaging (CT or MRI) at specified level (eg. L4)	Varies per study	Radiation exposure	Englesbe et al,[2] 2010 Tandon et al,[5] 2012 Montano-Loza et al,[56] 2014 Masuda & Shirabe,[10] 2014
	Bioimpedance analysis	Estimates amount of fat vs lean body mass	<90% of the standard skeletal muscle	Limited accuracy in patients with significant ascites	Kaido et al,[3] 2013
	Dual X-ray absorptiometry	Estimates skeletal muscle mass	<10th percentile based on age and gender	Radiation exposure	Figueiredo et al,[20] 2000 Peng et al,[16] 2007 Giusto et al,[21] 2015
	Jamar hand grip strength	Hand grip strength from dominant hand	<5th percentile based on age and gender	Limited in those with severe HE, interobserver variability	Figueiredo et al,[20] 2000 Huisman et al,[22] 2011 Giusto et al,[21] 2015
	Short Physical Performance Battery	Gait speed, repeat chair stands, tandem balance test	Score range from 0–12, varies per study	Limited in severe HE, ascites, edema	Lai et al,[6] 2014
	Gait Speed	Speed over 4–6 m	Speed <0.8 m/s	Limited in severe HE, ascites, edema	Lai et al,[6] 2014
	Get-up-and-go test	Time it takes to stand from a chair, walk a short distance, turn around, return and sit down	Score >3	Limited in severe HE, ascites, edema	—
	Anthropometry	1. Triceps skin-fold thickness 2. Mid-arm muscle circumference 3. BMI 4. Weight loss	<5th percentile <5th percentile <20 kg/m^2 ≥5%–10%	Interobserver variability	Kalaitzakis et al,[43] 2007 Merli et al,[57] 1996
	Subjective Global Assessment	Muscle wasting, fat loss, dietary intake, functional capacity	Severe muscle wasting and subcutaneous fat loss, inadequate dietary intake >5 wk, minimal functional capacity	Interobserver variability	Stephenson et al,[26] 2001

(continued on next page)

Table 1
(continued)

Syndrome	Disease Measure	Components	Abnormal Test Result Range	Considerations for Patients with Cirrhosis	Examples in the Literature
Frailty	Fried Frailty Index	Weight loss, exhaustion, weakness, slowness, and low levels of activity	Frailty score $\geq$3	Interobserver variability	Makary et al,[23] 2010 Lai et al,[6] 2014 McAdams-DeMarco et al,[34] 2015
	Cardiovascular Health Study Index	Weight loss >5%, weakness by grip strength, reduced energy level, slowness, low activity level	Score $\geq$3	Limited in severe HE, ascites, edema	Fried et al,[29] 2001 Ensrud et al,[30] 2008
	Rockwood Frailty Index	Number of health "deficits" that are manifest in the individual	Score $\geq$5	Limited in severe HE, ascites, edema	Rockwood et al,[31] 2005
	Study of Osteoporotic Fractures Frailty measure	Weight loss of >5%, inability to rise from a chair 5 times without using arms, reduced energy level	Score $\geq$2	Limited in severe HE, ascites, edema	Ensrud et al,[30] 2008

Abbreviations: BMI, body mass index; CT, computed tomography; HE, hepatic encephalopathy.

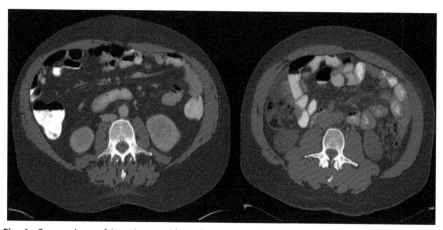

Fig. 1. Comparison of 2 patients with cirrhosis with identical BMI (32 kg/m²). Abdominal CT images taken at third lumbar vertebrae. Red color indicates skeletal muscles: rectus abdominis, oblique and lateral abdominal muscles, psoas, and paraspinal muscles. The patient on the left is sarcopenic with L3 skeletal muscle index of 49.82 cm²/m²; the patient on the right is not sarcopenic with L3 skeletal muscle index of 70.8 cm²/m². (*From* Montano-Loza AJ, Meza-Junco J, Prado CM, et al. Muscle wasting is associated with mortality in patients with cirrhosis. Clin Gastroenterol Hepatol 2012;10(2):169; with permission.)

dual X-ray absorptiometry, which incorporates X-rays at 2 different energy levels to separate bone from soft tissue and evaluates the ratio of low to high energy attenuation to separate body fat from lean body mass, has been used.[20,21] Although these imaging modalities lack a functional assessment of muscle strength, they have the advantages of being relatively easy to standardize, eliminating disease-specific confounders such as volume status and HE, and in many cases can be performed in retrospective studies to establish preliminary associations with clinical outcomes. However, the radiation exposure when computed tomography is used, the lack of high-quality prospective data comparing these methods, the limited availability of bioimpedance and absorptiometry testing, and the lack of functional assessment remain significant limitations of these radiographic approaches.

There are also several standardized approaches to measurement of muscle function that are available and can be used in combination with radiographic approaches. Hand grip strength (HGS), most often measured with devices such as the Jamar dynamometer, is among the most widely used.[20,22,23] HGS is sensitive, although less specific, for the identification of patients with protein-calorie malnutrition in cirrhosis.[20] In addition, tests that assess several muscle groups simultaneously or in series are also now validated in many groups, including the short physical performance battery[24] (repeated chair stands, balance testing, and walking speed), gait speed,[25] and the timed get-up-and-go test.[6,11] Although these physical tests offer a crucial functional assessment of the patient's muscular capabilities, they may be subject to interobserver variability and are likely to be more heavily influenced by disease-specific complications, including edema and HE.

Finally, tools such as the Subjective Global Assessment (SGA) have been used as a bedside method to identify patients with malnutrition and muscle depletion in cirrhosis.[20,22,26] Features of the SGA include presence of gastrointestinal symptoms and weight loss, dietary intake, and physical examination for fat, edema, and muscle wasting.[27]

Frailty

Frailty is defined by the American Geriatrics Society as a state of increased vulnerability to stressors due to age-related declines in physiologic reserve across neuromuscular, metabolic, and immune systems.[28] There are various measurement tools and indices that have been used to quantify frailty, including the Cardiovascular Health Study Index,[29] Fried Frailty Index,[23] the Study of Osteoporotic Fractures frailty measure,[30] and the Rockwood Frailty Index.[31] These tests collectively assess for weight loss, patient's energy level, and physical ability. They have been used as a risk assessment tool to identify those at highest risk of adverse outcomes and mortality, as well as to study the influence of frailty on particular diseases and interventions. Frailty has been studied extensively in patients with advanced age, cancer, human immunodeficiency virus infection, and in those who undergo various surgical interventions ranging from elective surgery to renal transplantation.[23,32–34]

The Fried Frailty Index, initially developed for assessment of patients older than 65 who had complications after elective surgery,[23] is now among the most widely used measures of frailty. The criteria include assessment in 5 key areas: weight loss, exhaustion, weakness, slowness, and low levels of physical activity (**Table 2**). Application of this scoring system to patients with advanced liver disease and HE may overestimate frailty, as this patient population is less likely to engage in physical activity and more apt to report exhaustion; however, this scale has now been used in studies evaluating morbidity and mortality in patients listed for liver transplantation.[6,35]

PATHOPHYSIOLOGY OF FRAILTY AND SARCOPENIA IN CIRRHOSIS

The pathogenesis of sarcopenia and frailty in patients with cirrhosis is multifactorial (**Box 1**, **Fig. 2**). There is an overall inadequate dietary intake to meet energy

Table 2
Components of the Fried Frailty Index

Testing Method	Criteria	Met Criteria for Frailty	Limitations in Patients with Cirrhosis
Shrinking	Unintentional weight loss	$\geq$10 pounds in the last year	Can be confounded by edema and ascites
Decreased grip strength (weakness)	Jamar hand grip strength	Lowest 20th percentile based on body mass index	Testing unlikely to be performed in severe hepatic encephalopathy
Exhaustion	Asked if everything was in effort	Moderate amount exhaustion during week	Subjective to patient
Low activity	Minnesota Leisure Time Activities Questionnaire	Lowest 20th percentile for activities for the week based on gender	Can be limited by large edema and ascites as well as hepatic encephalopathy
Slowed walking speed	Average of 3 trials of walking for 15 min	Lowest 20th percentile based on gender, height, weight	Can be limited by large edema and ascites as well as hepatic encephalopathy

From Makary MA, Segev DL, Pronovost PJ, et al. Frailty as a predictor of surgical outcomes in older patients. J Am Coll Surg 2010;210(6):903; with permission.

Box 1
Potential causes of sarcopenia in cirrhosis

Reduced caloric and protein intake

  Anorexia, gastroparesis, small intestinal dysmotility

  Ascites leading to early satiety

  Portal hypertension with impaired mucosal absorption

  Starvation related to procedures

  Dysgeusia

  Unpalatable diets due to salt restriction

Increased catabolism

  Hypermetabolism

  Sepsis

  Gastrointestinal bleeding

  Impaired protein synthesis response

  Insulin resistance

  Growth hormone deficiency

  Impaired signaling pathways in skeletal muscle

  Altered energy response with reduced plasma branched-chain amino acids

From Dasarathy J, Alkhouri N, Dasarathy S. Changes in body composition after transjugular intrahepatic portosystemic stent in cirrhosis: a critical review of literature. Liver Int 2011;31(9):1251; with permission.

---

expenditure. Patients with cirrhosis often have decreased appetite as a result of medications, HE, and ascites.[36] In addition, hormonal control of appetite may be altered. Patients with cirrhosis were found to have a twofold increase in leptin levels, an appetite-suppressing hormone, compared with healthy individuals.[15] There is also compromised nutrient absorption due to abnormal gut motility and diminished substrate utilization with impairment of glycogenolysis leading to gluconeogenesis via muscle breakdown. Finally, cirrhosis is associated with an increase in inflammatory cytokines resulting in a cytokine-driven hypermetabolic state, where the resting energy expenditure is 120% the expected value.[37] This cytokine-driven response may be further exacerbated by common complications of cirrhosis, including bleeding and infection.

In many cases, the underlying etiology of liver disease also plays a role in increased catabolism. The insulin resistance associated with nonalcoholic fatty liver disease impairs uptake of glucose and promotes gluconeogenesis via muscle breakdown.[15] Patients with alcohol-related liver disease often suffer from multiple nutritional deficiencies[37] and chronic viral hepatitis likely induces a chronic inflammatory state that could lead to decreased appetite and greater metabolic demands.[38]

Finally, studies also demonstrate reduced rates of whole body protein synthesis and increased rates of whole body protein breakdown in the postabsorptive state of patients with cirrhosis.[39] Patients are often in starvation mode, notably in the hospital while awaiting tests. During this time, amino acids are often broken down for gluconeogenesis, leading to decreased muscle mass.[37,40]

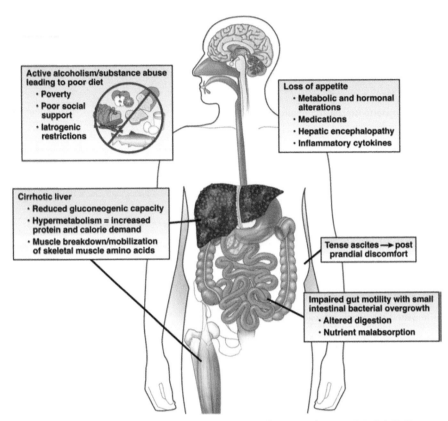

Fig. 2. Causes of decreased muscle mass in cirrhosis. (*From* Kachaamy T, Bajaj JS, Heuman DM. Muscle and mortality in cirrhosis. Clin Gastroenterol Hepatol 2012;10(2):100; with permission.)

INTERORGAN AMMONIA METABOLISM: PHYSIOLOGIC ASSOCIATION BETWEEN MUSCLE DEPLETION AND HEPATIC ENCEPHALOPATHY

Hyperammonemia remains central to the pathophysiology of HE. As a result, the altered ammonia metabolism seen in patients with cirrhosis and low muscle mass underlies the relationship between these clinical phenotypes. Multiple organs, prominently including the liver and skeletal muscle, are involved in the regulation of whole body ammonia homeostasis (**Fig. 3**).[41] In the normal state, arterial ammonia is tightly regulated to maintain plasma concentrations (10–40 μmol/L), but concentrations are in the mmol/L range in several organs including the intestine and kidney, which are also key regulators of total body ammonia. Ammonia metabolism and concentrations in each organ are largely dependent on a balance in the conversion of ammonia to glutamine, a nonessential amino acid that constitutes a significant portion of the total body amino acids. Ammonia and glutamate are converted to glutamine by glutamate synthetase (GS), and the reciprocal reaction converting glutamine to ammonia and glutamate is carried out by phosphate-activated glutaminase (PAG).

In healthy patients, the liver is the main site of metabolism of dietary proteins. Periportal hepatocytes play a key role in the urea cycle, which converts ammonia to urea, the major end-product of nitrogen metabolism, which is excreted by the kidney.

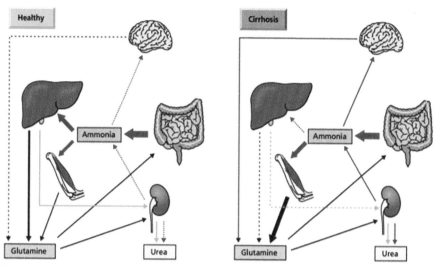

Fig. 3. Comparison of ammonia metabolism and detoxification in patients without (*left*) and with cirrhosis (*right*). The red arrows represent ammonia, the black arrows represent glutamine, and the green arrows represent urea. In healthy individuals, the liver converts ammonia into urea, which is excreted by the kidneys. In patients with cirrhosis, ammonia is metabolized mainly in skeletal muscle and is then excreted in the kidney. Because the liver is impaired, the resulting glutamine is often synthesized back into ammonia in the gut and the cycle continues. (*From* Morgan MY. Hepatic encephalopathy in patients with cirrhosis. In: Dooley JS, Lok AS, Burroughs AK, editors. Sherlock's diseases of the liver and biliary system. 12th edition. Chichester, UK: Blackwell Publishing Ltd; 2011. p. 145; with permission.)

However, these cells also have significant PAG activity to provide the glutamate required for urea cycle function. Conversely, peri-venous hepatocytes have abundant GS,[42] which detoxifies the ammonia that has passed through the peri-portal region. Thus, hepatic glutamine metabolism and urea cycle function are central to the regulation of systemic ammonia levels.

In addition to the liver, normal total body ammonia levels are regulated by enzyme activity in (1) the gut, a significant source of ammonia from dietary nitrogen as well as through conversion of glutamine to ammonia as its major source of energy; (2) the kidneys, which are essential for ammonia excretion; (3) the brain, where ammonia is central to glial cell metabolism, and is converted to glutamine and then to important neurotransmitters; and (4) skeletal muscle. In skeletal muscle, although GS activity may be relatively low, the total mass of skeletal muscle in the body renders this pathway crucial to ammonia metabolism with significant conversion to glutamine. This glutamine can then be excreted by the kidneys; however, it also may be taken up by enterocytes to again produce ammonia, continuing this cycle.[43]

In the setting of advanced cirrhosis and portal hypertension, hepatocyte loss and portal-systemic shunting reduce the capacity of the liver to detoxify ammonia. Consequently, there is an increased need for alternative pathways of ammonia metabolism and clearance. Ammonia metabolism is altered in several organs in the setting of liver dysfunction. Intestinal PAG activity is fourfold higher in patients with cirrhosis compared with healthy controls.[8,44] In addition, a net increase in ammonia may be seen because of increased renal ammonia production and decreased excretion in patients with advanced liver disease. This net increase in renal ammonia production may be particularly pronounced in patients with decreased renal perfusion due to diuretics or splanchnic vasodilation and hepatorenal syndrome.[45–47] Therefore, skeletal muscle becomes a crucial alternative pathway for the metabolism and breakdown of ammonia in the setting of advanced liver disease, and it has been postulated for some time that patients with cirrhosis with significant muscle wasting are at high risk of hyperammonemia.[48–52]

In addition to this essential relationship between muscle mass and ammonia metabolism, the muscle protein catabolism that is prevalent in cirrhosis leads to increased glutamine release from muscle, which is converted to ammonia by the intestine and kidney. Finally, hyperammonemia may itself promote muscle breakdown, leading to sarcopenia and HE through the direct regulation of myostatin production, an inhibitor of skeletal muscle growth.[39] This mechanism has been demonstrated in murine models, where hyperammonemia was found to induce transcriptional regulation of myostatin by NF-κβ.[53] Murine models have also shown that hyperammonemia induces skeletal muscle autophagy and further breakdown of proteins to provide nutrients.[54]

THE IMPACT OF SARCOPENIA AND FRAILTY ON THE RISK OF HEPATIC ENCEPHALOPATHY
Sarcopenia and Increased Risk of Hepatic Encephalopathy

Sarcopenia and frailty are thus important predictors of HE and are often underrecognized comorbid conditions (**Table 3**). This has been demonstrated in several studies, including by Merli and colleagues[13] who enrolled 300 consecutive patients and evaluated the relationship between nutritional status and HE. Mid-arm muscle circumference and triceps skin-fold thickness were assessed as measures of sarcopenia. The prevalence of overt HE was higher in patients with muscle depletion and decreased muscle strength, and venous blood ammonia levels also were higher with those who had sarcopenia. Protein malnutrition was found to have an odds ratio of 3.4 for predicting the presence of overt HE. In addition, Kalaitzakis and colleagues[43] studied 128 patients with cirrhosis and found that sarcopenia, defined by triceps skin-fold thickness and mid-arm muscle circumference in the lowest fifth percentile compared with the standard population, predicted the presence of HE. Forty-six percent of patients with sarcopenia had HE defined by the West Haven criteria versus 27% without protein malnutrition. Sarcopenia was found to be an independent risk factor for HE when adjusted for age, Child-Pugh score, and the presence of diabetes mellitus.

Poor muscle function as evaluated by functional testing such as HGS also has been associated with an increased prevalence of HE. In a prospective study of 84 patients, 29% with low HGS had HE compared with none of the patients with normal grip strength.[22]

However, not all studies have confirmed this association between sarcopenia and HE, perhaps in part a result of the patient population studied and the definitions used.[55] Montano-Loza and colleagues[56] evaluated sarcopenia by skeletal muscle index at the third lumbar vertebra, and found that 45% of 248 patients undergoing liver transplantation met criteria for sarcopenia. After a median follow-up of 39 months, there was more encephalopathy in the sarcopenic group (60% vs 49%, $P = .10$); however, this difference was not statistically significant. A significant difference in mortality was seen only in men in the lowest sextile for sarcopenia (median survival 71 vs 132 months), but otherwise there was no significant correlation between sarcopenia and mortality. It is possible that this study overestimated the prevalence of sarcopenia based on the investigators' definition, as those in the lowest sextile were the only patients with a significant mortality difference.

Frailty and Increased Risk of Hepatic Encephalopathy

A recent prospective study was the first to apply clinical measures of frailty to a liver transplant cohort (see **Table 3**).[6] In this study, 294 outpatients with Model for End Stage Liver Disease (MELD) score of $\geq$12 on the transplant list underwent 4 frailty assessments, including the Fried Frailty Index. They were then divided into frail (score $\geq$3) or not frail and followed for a median of 12 months. Moderate HE (defined as Numbers Connection Test score between 60 and 120 seconds) was more prevalent in the frail patients (26%) compared with those who were not classified as frail (17%), although this difference did not reach statistical significance (P = .17). However, patients with severe HE (Numbers Connection Test score >120 seconds) were excluded from the study (highlighting a major limitation to studying this association) and the overall number of frail patients was relatively small. A similar numerical difference was seen in a smaller cohort of 82 patients on the transplant wait list evaluated with the Fried Frailty Index, in which 65% of frail patients had a history of overt HE compared with 46% of controls (P = .10).[35]

THE IMPACT OF FRAILTY AND SARCOPENIA ON MORTALITY IN CIRRHOSIS

There is a clear association between frailty, sarcopenia, and mortality in cirrhosis. In one of the largest studies of sarcopenia in cirrhosis, mid-arm fat area was used in a prospective study of 1053 patients with cirrhosis in a multicenter trial. Patients were defined as having malnourishment or sarcopenia if the mid-arm muscle area or mid-arm fat area was below the fifth percentile in a population matched for age and sex. With a median of 3 years of follow-up, sarcopenia had a relative risk of 1.79 for mortality in unadjusted analysis, although it was not found to be an independent risk factor when controlling for age, sex, bilirubin, ascites, and varices.[57]

Imaging measures of sarcopenia also have been associated with increased mortality risk on patients with cirrhosis. The skeletal muscle index,[17] defined as the cross-sectional area of muscle and adipose tissue normalized for stature at the L3 spine level, was evaluated in a cohort of 112 patients with cirrhosis.[18] Using a cutoff of $\leq$38.5 cm^2/m^2 for women and $\leq$52.4 cm^2/m^2 for men, 40% of the patients were found to be sarcopenic and to have lower BMIs. The median survival of patients with low skeletal muscle index was 19 versus 34 months in those with a normal muscle index. Sarcopenia was an independent risk factor for mortality when adjusted for ascites, encephalopathy, creatinine, bilirubin, and albumin (hazard ratio 2.18, P = .006). A similar study defining sarcopenia as greater than two standard deviations below normal in the cross-sectional area of 5 muscle groups at the L3 level also found sarcopenia predictive of mortality in patients on the transplant wait list.[5]

Imaging of the psoas muscle area also has been used to prognosticate mortality in patients with cirrhosis,[58,59] as well as those undergoing liver transplantation.[4] More recently a review of psoas muscle thickness suggested that a MELD-psoas score was better than the MELD score or MELD-Na score in prognosticating mortality.[60] Unfortunately, HE was not examined in these studies, as they were mainly retrospective and focused on imaging for prognosis.

Finally, in the aforementioned study looking at mortality on the transplant wait list, 22% of frail patients by the Fried Frailty Index versus 10% of not-frail patients died or were delisted for being too sick.[6] There was a larger discrepancy if the MELD score was less than 18, as 23% of the frail cohort versus 9% of the not-frail cohort died or were delisted, suggesting that the frail population is underserved by the MELD score and has a higher mortality while waiting for liver transplantation.

Table 3
The impact of sarcopenia and frailty on the risk of HE

Study	Patient Population	Diagnostic Test	Components	Range of Normal/ Abnormal	Prevalence of Sarcopenia or Frailty	Relation to HE
Kalaitzakis et al,[43] 2007	128 patients with cirrhosis	Anthropometry	1. Triceps skin-fold thickness 2. Mid-arm muscle circumference 3. BMI 4. Weight loss	<5th percentile <5th percentile <20 kg/m² ≥5%–10%	40%	HE in 46% with malnutrition vs 27% without malnutrition ($P = .03$)
Huisman et al,[22] 2011	84 patients with cirrhosis	Jamar hand grip strength	Hand grip strength in dominant hand	<5th percentile based on age and gender	67%	HE in 29% with malnutrition vs 0% without malnutrition ($P < .01$)
Meza-Junco et al,[17] 2013	116 patients with HCC being evaluated for liver transplant	Skeletal muscle mass at third lumbar spine	Cross-sectional area	≤41 cm²/m² for women <53 cm²/m² for men	35%	HE in 23% with sarcopenia vs 12% without sarcopenia ($P = .2$)
Merli et al,[13] 2013	300 patients with cirrhosis	Anthropometry	Mid-arm-muscle circumference Handgrip strength	<5th percentile <5th percentile	48%	Overt HE in 30% with sarcopenia vs 15% without sarcopenia ($P = .003$) Minimal HE in 49% with sarcopenia vs 30% without sarcopenia ($P = .001$)

Montano-Loza et al,[56] 2014	248 patients with cirrhosis undergoing OLT	3rd lumbar spine area	Cross-sectional area of muscle and adipose tissue normalized for stature	<41 cm²/m² for women, <53 cm²/m² for men	45%	HE in 60% with sarcopenia vs 49% without sarcopenia ($P = .10$)
Verna et al,[35] 2014	82 patients on the LT wait list	Fried Frailty Instrument	Presence of gait speed, exhaustion, physical activity, unintentional weight loss, weakness	Frailty ≥3 variables	38%	HE in 65% of frail patients vs 46% who were not frail ($P = .10$)
Lai et al,[6] 2014	294 patients on the LT wait list	Fried Frailty Instrument	Presence of gait speed, exhaustion, physical activity, unintentional weight loss, weakness	Frailty ≥3 variables	17%	HE in 26% of frail patients vs 17% who were not frail ($P = .17$)

Abbreviations: BMI, body mass index; HCC, hepatocellular carcinoma; HE, hepatic encephalopathy; LT, liver transplantation; OLT, orthotopic liver transplantation.

FRAILTY AND SARCOPENIA IN LIVER TRANSPLANT RECIPIENTS

One in 5 patients on the waiting list will die or become too sick for liver transplantation.[6] Patients with cirrhosis with frailty tend to have increased rates of mortality before and after liver transplantation.[10,57] Despite this, there are no standardized objective parameters that institutions use when determining criteria for delisting or a decision not to list patients for transplantation. Frailty, however, remains one of the primary contraindications to liver transplant listing and a frequently cited reason for delisting. Patients who are delisted for being too frail often have significant HE but do not have the highest MELD scores, suggesting that there is an unaccounted risk of adverse outcome due to frailty that is not captured by the MELD score. This risk has been demonstrated as patients with sarcopenia have worse outcomes after liver transplantation.[3,5,10]

For example, in a study by Englesbe and colleagues,[2] pretransplant sarcopenia as defined by psoas muscle area was associated with increased post transplant mortality. Psoas area was calculated retrospectively from perioperative abdominal imaging in 163 patients undergoing liver transplantation. Although the total psoas area correlated poorly with MELD score, it was strongly associated with posttransplant mortality with a hazard ratio of 3.7 for every 1000 mm^2 decrease in psoas area muscle. Those patients in the lowest quartile of psoas area also were found to have only a 27% 3-month survival after liver transplantation. In addition, in a cohort of 124 living donor liver transplant recipients, skeletal muscle mass as measured by a body composition analyzer was significantly predictive of survival after liver transplantation.[3] Another cohort of 200 living donor liver transplant recipients revealed that high intramuscular adipose content (odds ratio 3.9, 95% confidence interval 2.0–7.8, $P<.001$) and low psoas muscle index (odds ratio 3.6, 95% confidence interval 1.9–7.2, $P<.001$) were independently predictive of mortality after liver transplantation.[4] Malnutrition and sarcopenia may also specifically increase the risk of complications after liver transplantation, including infection,[61] the need for blood transfusion, and longer hospital stays.[26]

In our center, 82 patients with cirrhosis listed for transplantation were examined prospectively for elements of frailty.[35] Patients who were deemed to be frail by the Fried Frailty Index had a higher incidence of a composite outcome of post-transplant death, re-operation or infection (66% in frail patients vs 26% in nonfrail patients, $P = .008$). In this cohort, physical measures such as walk speed and the short physical performance battery were the most predictive of important clinical outcomes, including pre–liver transplantation and overall mortality.

MANAGEMENT OF FRAILTY AND SARCOPENIA IN PATIENTS WITH CIRRHOSIS AND HEPATIC ENCEPHALOPATHY
Nutrition

The pathophysiologic link between sarcopenia and HE is also suggested by the efficacy of nutritional interventions in the treatment of both syndromes. Malnutrition is among the most common complications of cirrhosis, with a prevalence as high as 65% to 90%,[61] yet often goes unrecognized given the complexities of this assessment in patients with ascites or who are at baseline overweight. As described previously, protein-calorie malnutrition in cirrhosis is likely the result of multiple coinciding factors, including the catabolic state of chronic liver disease, poor dietary intake that is inadequate to meet energy expenditure, compromised absorption, and diminished substrate utilization in the setting of impaired liver function. This malnutrition is inherently linked to the pathogenesis of hepatic encephalopathy as glutamine broken down in the muscle becomes converted to ammonia and contributes to HE. Thus, nutrition clearly plays a pivotal role in management of frailty, sarcopenia, and HE.

Key targets to combat muscle depletion in this setting include reducing the time between meals and increasing total caloric and protein intake, with the aim to decrease gluconeogenesis and increase muscle mass.[9] Diets that include small frequent meals and nighttime snacks have been shown to prevent lipid and muscle catabolism, leading to less ammonia production and HE.[15,62] Nocturnal supplements also have been suggested, as they reduce gluconeogenesis and therefore protein catabolism.[15,39] In a study by Plank and colleagues,[63] 103 patients with cirrhosis were randomized to either daytime or nighttime supplementary nutrition of 710 kcal per day. There was a significant improvement in total body protein and fat-free mass in the patients who received nocturnal supplementation, but the study was limited by high dropout rate and nonadherence with taking the supplement at the correct time.

It was previously thought that a high-protein diet leads to worsening HE,[64] and it remains relevant that feeding does increase intestinal ammonia generation, particularly with ingestion of animal protein.[65] However, it is now known that patients with cirrhosis may in fact have increased protein requirements,[66] and that increased protein intake may lead to increased protein synthesis[67] and maintenance or restoration of muscle mass. It was not until 1997 that the European Guidelines recommended higher protein requirements of 1.2 g/kg per day based on studies evaluating nutrition in patients with alcoholic hepatitis,[68] and this diet is now recommended by joint society guidelines.[69] When studied prospectively, a high-calorie–high-protein diet consisting of vegetable-based and milk-based proteins, as well as a nighttime snack, led to improvement in HE in 80% of patients admitted with overt encephalopathy.[70] Though this trial did not include a control group, all of the patients had improvements in their ammonia levels, debunking the association between high protein intake and HE.

A recent Cochrane review[71] analyzed the impact of numerous dietary interventions and supplements on outcomes in cirrhosis, and 12 studies were noted to have assessed the impact of dietary interventions on HE in particular.[72,73] Among the 2 prospective trials for treatment of HE in hospitalized patients, the administration of branched-chain amino acid (BCAA) supplementation was significantly associated with clearance of HE. BCAAs are essential for protein synthesis and regulation of energy metabolism leading to anticatabolic effects[15,74] and plasma levels of BCAAs are often low in the setting of cirrhosis. In addition, hyperammonemia leads to skeletal muscle BCAA metabolism,[75] thus there is interest in BCAA supplementation in these patients. However, BCAA also may transiently increase ammonia levels in patients with cirrhosis, as they are metabolized to glutamine, which is reabsorbed by enterocytes to form ammonia.[76] Despite this risk, BCAA use has been shown to improve event-free survival and quality of life in patients with cirrhosis.[58,77,78] In addition, a more recent meta-analysis of 8 studies (n = 382 total) demonstrated improvement in HE with a risk ratio of 1.71 (95% confidence interval 1.17–2.51) and a number needed to treat of 5 patients.[79] Although there are limitations in the palatability and cost of BCAA formulations, they could play a future role in those patients with sarcopenia and HE. BCAAs are now recognized for their potential in patients with HE by the most recent multisociety practice guidelines.[69]

Other Future Treatment Options

Several medical interventions are now used to target hyperammonemia due to urea cycle deficiencies and inborn errors of metabolism, but have not been widely used in adult patients with decompensated cirrhosis and HE. These medical therapies include phenylbutyrate, which is converted to phenylacetate in vivo and binds circulating glutamine to form phenylacetylglutamine, which is excreted by the kidneys. Glycerol phenylbutyrate was recently tested in a randomized controlled trial of patients with 2 or more previous episodes of HE in the previous 6 months, and treatment was associated with fewer episodes of HE and hospitalizations.[80] In addition, L-ornithine and L-aspartate, amino acid substrates for glutamine production in muscle and elsewhere, also has been studied and may have some efficacy in the treatment of HE in the intravenous form,[81] although with the concern that the increased glutamine may become a source for rebound hyperammonemia through production in the intestine and kidneys. However, a novel agent that targets this complex interorgan relationship and combines the benefits of these 2 approaches, L-ornithine phenylacetate, has recently been developed. This compound both detoxifies ammonia to glutamine and promotes renal glutamine excretion rather than ammonia regeneration. L-ornithine phenylacetate has now been studied with promising results in animal models,[82,83] may have an acceptable safety profile in humans,[84] and studies are ongoing for the treatment of HE associated with both cirrhosis and acute liver failure.

Myostatin, a growth factor that inhibits muscle differentiation, may be elevated in the patient with cirrhosis compared with controls without liver disease.[85] Follistatin, a myostatin antagonist, has been shown in animal studies to improve skeletal muscle mass and may be of interest in studying in patients with cirrhosis-related sarcopenia and HE. Using a rat model of sarcopenia with a portocaval anastomosis, phenylalanine was used to quantify the fractional and absolute protein synthesis rates in skeletal muscle.[86] Protein synthesis was found to be decreased in those with a portocaval anastomosis. Follistatin was then administered to assess for proliferation of myocyte precursors. Portocaval anastomosis rats that were treated with follistatin had significantly greater weight gain (372 vs 274 g) and gastrocnemius muscle size (1.5 vs 0.93 g). Follistatin also led to increased grip strength in this murine study compared with placebo, suggesting a possible treatment opportunity for human trials that have yet to be studied.

Transjugular intrahepatic portosystemic shunt (TIPS) placement also has been suggested as a potential therapy for sarcopenia. Although TIPS worsens shunting and hyperammonemia, and therefore may worsen HE, it can also decrease risk of variceal bleeding and improve portal hypertension, potentially leading to improved gut motility and nutrient absorption as well as increased appetite by reducing ascites. Two small prospective studies demonstrated an increase in muscle mass after TIPS placement.[87,88] Others have shown that TIPS increases adiponectin production, suggesting a greater anabolic state.[19] It is not known whether in the long term, restoration of muscle mass before the development of overt HE may ameliorate the worsened hyperammonemia seen due to shunting in the early post-TIPS period. At this time, TIPS cannot be recommended for this indication.

Finally, there are limited data regarding the effect of exercise and intensive rehabilitation on outcomes in patients with liver disease.[62] A pilot study revealed improvement in a 6-minute walk test in those who combined daily leucine supplementations with hour-long treadmill and cycle exercise 3 times a week with to achieve 60% to 70% maximum heart rate.[89] In this randomized pilot study, 17 patients with cirrhosis were randomized to a treatment arm consisting of 12 weeks of exercise, or control. At the 24-week follow-up, patients who exercised had a significant increase in thigh muscle circumference and in overall weight. Plasma ammonia levels decreased in both groups; however, HE was not examined in this study. The role of exercise in the treatment of HE has not been explored and may be difficult in patients with overt HE and/or significant extracellular volume expansion. However, disease-specific modifications to the recommended exercise routines may help to overcome some of these limitations.

SUMMARY

Normal regulation of total body and circulating ammonia requires a delicate interplay in ammonia formation and breakdown between several organ systems. In the setting of cirrhosis and portal hypertension, the decreased hepatic clearance of ammonia leads to significant dependence on skeletal muscle for ammonia detoxification; however, cirrhosis is also associated with muscle depletion and decreased functional muscle mass. Thus, patients with diminished muscle mass and sarcopenia may have a decreased ability to compensate for hepatic insufficiency and a higher likelihood of developing physiologically significant hyperammonemia and HE.

Although there are currently no cirrhosis-specific measures of sarcopenia and frailty, the available data indicate that these syndromes are highly prevalent in cirrhosis and predict important clinical outcomes, including mortality, often independent of traditional predictors such as MELD. In addition, the clinical relationship among sarcopenia, frailty, and HE has been explored, and additional investigation into this physiologic relationship may point to novel therapeutic targets, including nutritional, pharmacologic, and perhaps physical interventions. Some currently used frailty assessments are not possible in patients with severe HE and therefore focusing on more objective, imaging-based tests, such as psoas muscle area, may be better suited to quantify sarcopenia in this population. It remains unknown whether reversal of sarcopenia may improve hyperammonemia and thus prevent the development or recurrence of HE, but this relationship may be an important target for additional study.

REFERENCES

1. Waits S, Kim EK, Terjimanian MN, et al. Morphometric age and mortality after liver transplant. JAMA Surg 2014;149(4):335–40.
2. Englesbe MJ, Patel SP, He K, et al. Sarcopenia and mortality after liver transplantation. J Am Coll Surg 2010;211(2):271–8.
3. Kaido T, Ogawa K, Fujimoto Y. Impact of sarcopenia on survival in patients undergoing living donor liver transplantation. Am J Transplant 2013;13:1549–56.
4. Hamaguchi Y, Kaido T, Okumura S, et al. Impact of quality as well as quantity of skeletal muscle on outcomes after liver transplantation. Liver Transpl 2014;20:1413–9.
5. Tandon P, Ney M, Irwin I. Severe muscle depletion in patients on the liver transplant wait list: its prevalence and independent prognostic value. Liver Transpl 2012;18:1209–16.
6. Lai JC, Feng S, Terrault N, et al. Frailty predicts waitlist mortality in liver transplant candidates. Am J Transplant 2014;14(8):1870–9.
7. Bajaj J-S. Minimal hepatic encephalopathy matters in daily life. World J Gastroenterol 2008;14(23):3609–15.
8. Morgan MY. Hepatic encephalopathy in patients with cirrhosis. In: Dooley JS, Lok AS, Burroughs AK, et al, editors. Sherlock's diseases of the liver and biliary system. 12th edition. Chichester, UK: Blackwell Publishing Ltd; 2011. p. 121–51.
9. Periyalwar P, Dasarathy S. Malnutrition in cirrhosis: contribution and consequences of sarcopenia on metabolic and clinical responses. Clin Liver Dis 2012;16(1):95–131.
10. Masuda T, Shirabe K. Sarcopenia is a prognostic factor in living donor liver transplantation. Liver Transpl 2014;20:401–7.
11. Cruz-Jentoft AJ, Baeyens JP, Bauer JM, et al. Sarcopenia: European consensus on definition and diagnosis: report of the European Working Group on sarcopenia in older people. Age Ageing 2010;39(4):412–23.

12. Lang P-O, Michel J-P, Zekry D. Frailty syndrome: a transitional state in a dynamic process. Gerontology 2009;55(5):539–49.

13. Merli M, Giusto M, Lucidi C, et al. Muscle depletion increases the risk of overt and minimal hepatic encephalopathy: results of a prospective study. Metab Brain Dis 2013;28(2):281–4.

14. Selberg O, Bottcher J, Tusch G. Identification of high- and low-risk patients before liver transplantation: a prospective cohort study of nutritional and metabolic parameters in 150 patients. Hepatology 1997;25:652–7.

15. Cheung K, Lee SS, Raman M. Prevalence and mechanisms of malnutrition in patients with advanced liver disease, and nutrition management strategies. Clin Gastroenterol Hepatol 2012;10(2):117–25.

16. Peng S, Plank LD, Mccall JL, et al. Body composition, muscle function, and energy expenditure in patients with liver cirrhosis: a comprehensive study. Am J Clin Nutr 2007;85:1257–66.

17. Meza-Junco J, Montano-Loza AJ, Baracos VE, et al. Sarcopenia as a prognostic index of nutritional status in concurrent cirrhosis and hepatocellular carcinoma. J Clin Gastroenterol 2013;47(10):861–70.

18. Montano-Loza AJ, Meza-Junco J, Prado CM, et al. Muscle wasting is associated with mortality in patients with cirrhosis. Clin Gastroenterol Hepatol 2012;10(2): 166–73, 173.e1.

19. Thomsen KL, Sandahl TD, Holland-Fischer P, et al. Changes in adipokines after transjugular intrahepatic porto-systemic shunt indicate an anabolic shift in metabolism. Clin Nutr 2012;31(6):940–5.

20. Figueiredo FA, Dickson ER, Pasha TM, et al. Utility of standard nutritional parameters in detecting body cell mass depletion in patients with end-stage liver disease. Liver Transpl 2000;6(5):575–81.

21. Giusto M, Lattanzi B, Albanese C, et al. Sarcopenia in liver cirrhosis: the role of computed tomography scan for the assessment of muscle mass compared with dual-energy X-ray absorptiometry and anthropometry. Eur J Gastroenterol Hepatol 2015;27(3):328–34.

22. Huisman EJ, Trip EJ, Siersema PD, et al. Protein energy malnutrition predicts complications in liver cirrhosis. Eur J Gastroenterol Hepatol 2011;23(11):982–9.

23. Makary MA, Segev DL, Pronovost PJ, et al. Frailty as a predictor of surgical outcomes in older patients. J Am Coll Surg 2010;210(6):901–8.

24. Guralnik JM, Simonsick EM, Ferrucci L, et al. A short physical performance battery assessing lower extremity function: association with self-reported disability and prediction of mortality and nursing home admission. J Gerontol 1994; 49(2):85–94.

25. Buchner DM, Larson EB, Wagner EH, et al. Evidence for a non-linear relationship between leg strength and gait speed. Age Ageing 1996;25:386–91.

26. Stephenson G, Moretti E, El-Moalem H, et al. Malnutrition in liver transplant patients: preoperative subjective global assessment is predictive of outcome after liver transplantation. Transplantation 2001;72(4):666–70.

27. Montano-Loza AJ. Clinical relevance of sarcopenia in patients with cirrhosis. World J Gastroenterol 2014;20(25):8061–71.

28. Walston J, Hadley EC, Ferrucci L, et al. Research agenda for frailty in older adults: toward a better understanding of physiology and etiology: summary from the American Geriatrics Society/National Institute on Aging Research Conference on Frailty in Older Adults. J Am Geriatr Soc 2006;54(6):991–1001.

29. Fried LP, Tangen CM, Walston J, et al. Frailty in older adults: evidence for a phenotype. J Gerontol A Biol Sci Med Sci 2001;56(3):146–57.

30. Ensrud KE, Ewing SK, Taylor BC, et al. Comparison of 2 frailty indexes for prediction of falls, disability, fractures, and death in older women. Arch Intern Med 2008; 168(4):382–9.
31. Rockwood K, Song X, Macknight C, et al. A global clinical measure of fitness and frailty in elderly people. Can Med Assoc J 2005;173(5):489–95.
32. Ensrud KE, Ewing SK, Cawthon PM, et al. A comparison of frailty indexes for the prediction of falls, disability, fractures and mortality in older men. J Am Geriatr Soc 2010;57(3):492–8.
33. Brothers TD, Kirkland S, Guaraldi G, et al. Frailty in people aging with human immunodeficiency virus (HIV) infection. J Infect Dis 2014;210(8):1170–9.
34. McAdams-DeMarco MA, Law A, King E, et al. Frailty and mortality in kidney transplant recipients. Am J Transplant 2015;15(1):149–54.
35. Verna E, Chan C, Pisa J, et al. Frailty, physical performance, and sarcopenia measures in patients awaiting liver transplantation predict mortality and postoperative complications. Am J Transplant 2014;14(S3):742.
36. Kachaamy T, Bajaj JS, Heuman DM. Muscle and mortality in cirrhosis. Clin Gastroenterol Hepatol 2012;10(2):100–2.
37. Tsiaousi ET, Hatzitolios AI, Trygonis SK, et al. Malnutrition in end stage liver disease: recommendations and nutritional support. J Gastroenterol Hepatol 2008; 23(4):527–33.
38. Gowda C, Compher C, Amorosa VK, et al. Association between chronic hepatitis C virus infection and low muscle mass in US adults. J Viral Hepat 2014;21(12): 938–43.
39. Tsien CD, McCullough AJ, Dasarathy S. Late evening snack: exploiting a period of anabolic opportunity in cirrhosis. J Gastroenterol Hepatol 2012;27(3):430–41.
40. Ghany MG, Nelson DR, Strader DB, et al. An update on treatment of genotype 1 chronic hepatitis C virus infection: 2011 practice guideline by the American Association for the Study of Liver Diseases. Hepatology 2011;54(4):1433–44.
41. Wright G, Noiret L, Olde Damink SW, et al. Interorgan ammonia metabolism in liver failure: the basis of current and future therapies. Liver Int 2011;31(2): 163–75.
42. Gebhardt R, Mecke D. Heterogeneous distribution of glutamine synthetase parenchymal cells in situ and in primary culture. EMBO J 1983;2(4):567–70.
43. Kalaitzakis E, Olsson R, Henfridsson P, et al. Malnutrition and diabetes mellitus are related to hepatic encephalopathy in patients with liver cirrhosis. Liver Int 2007;27(9):1194–201.
44. Romero-Gómez M, Ramos-Guerrero R, Grande L, et al. Intestinal glutaminase activity is increased in liver cirrhosis and correlates with minimal hepatic encephalopathy. J Hepatol 2004;41(1):49–54.
45. Jalan R, Kapoor D. Enhanced renal ammonia excretion following volume expansion in patients with well compensated cirrhosis of the liver. Gut 2003;52(7): 1041–5.
46. Owen E, Tyor M, Flanagan J, et al. The kidney as a source of blood ammonia in patients with liver disease: the effect of acetazolamide. J Clin Invest 1960;39: 288–94.
47. Olde Damink SW, Jalan R, Deutz NE, et al. The kidney plays a major role in the hyperammonemia seen after simulated or actual GI bleeding in patients with cirrhosis. Hepatology 2003;37(6):1277–85.
48. Olde Damink SW, Jalan R, Redhead DN, et al. Interorgan ammonia and amino acid metabolism in metabolically stable patients with cirrhosis and a TIPSS. Hepatology 2002;36(5):1163–71.

49. Ganda O, Ruderman N. Muscle nitrogen metabolism in chronic hepatic insufficiency. Metabolism 1976;25(4):427–35.
50. Bessman S, Bradley J. Uptake of ammonia by muscle; its implications in ammoniagenic coma. N Engl J Med 2015;253(26):1143–7.
51. Tyor M, Owen E, Berry J, et al. The relative role of extremity, liver, and kidney as ammonia receivers and donors in patients with liver disease. Gastroenterology 1960;39:420–4.
52. Bessman S, Bessman A. The cerebral and peripheral uptake of ammonia in liver disease with an hypothesis for the mechanism of coma. J Clin Invest 1954;34(4): 622–8.
53. Qiu J, Thapaliya S, Runkana A, et al. Hyperammonemia in cirrhosis induces transcriptional regulation of myostatin by an NF-κB-mediated mechanism. Proc Natl Acad Sci U S A 2013;110(45):18162–7.
54. Qiu J, Tsien C, Thapalaya S, et al. Hyperammonemia-mediated autophagy in skeletal muscle contributes to sarcopenia of cirrhosis. Am J Physiol Endocrinol Metab 2012;303(8):E983–93.
55. Sörös P, Böttcher J, Weissenborn K, et al. Malnutrition and hypermetabolism are not risk factors for the presence of hepatic encephalopathy: a cross-sectional study. J Gastroenterol Hepatol 2008;23(4):606–10.
56. Montano-Loza AJ, Meza-Junco J, Baracos VE, et al. Severe muscle depletion predicts postoperative length of stay but is not associated with survival after liver transplantation. Liver Transpl 2014;20:640–8.
57. Merli M, Riggio O, Dally L. Does malnutrition affect survival in cirrhosis? Hepatology 1996;23:1041–6.
58. Hanai T, Shiraki M, Nishimura K, et al. Sarcopenia impairs prognosis of patients with liver cirrhosis. Nutrition 2015;31(1):193–9.
59. Kim TY, Kim MY, Sohn JH, et al. Sarcopenia as a useful predictor for long-term mortality in cirrhotic patients with ascites. J Korean Med Sci 2014;29: 1253–9.
60. Durand F, Buyse S, Francoz C, et al. Prognostic value of muscle atrophy in cirrhosis using psoas muscle thickness on computed tomography. J Hepatol 2014;60(6):1151–7.
61. Merli M, Giusto M, Gentili F, et al. Nutritional status: its influence on the outcome of patients undergoing liver transplantation. Liver Int 2010;30(2):208–14.
62. Toshikuni N, Arisawa T, Tsutsumi M. Nutrition and exercise in the management of liver cirrhosis. World J Gastroenterol 2014;20(23):7286–97.
63. Plank LD, Gane EJ, Peng S, et al. Nocturnal nutritional supplementation improves total body protein status of patients with liver cirrhosis: a randomized 12-month trial. Hepatology 2008;48(2):557–66.
64. Sherlock S, Summerskill W, White L, et al. Portal-systemic encephalopathy neurological complications of liver disease. Lancet 1954;267:454–7.
65. Rudman D, Galambos J, Smith R, et al. Comparison of the effect of various amino acids upon the blood ammonia concentration patients with liver disease. Am J Clin Nutr 1973;26(9):916–25.
66. Swart G, van den Berg J, Wattimena J, et al. Elevated protein requirements in cirrhosis of the liver investigated by whole body protein turnover studies. Clin Sci 1988;75(1):101–7.
67. Kondrup J, Nielsen K, Juul A. Effect of long-term refeeding on protein metabolism in patients with cirrhosis of the liver. Br J Nutr 1996;77(2):197–212.
68. Plauth M, Cabré E, Riggio O, et al. ESPEN guidelines on enteral nutrition: liver disease. Clin Nutr 2006;25(2):285–94.

69. Vilstrup H, Amodio P, Bajaj J, et al. Hepatic encephalopathy in chronic liver disease: 2014 practice guideline by the American Association for the Study of Liver Diseases and the European Association for the Study of the Liver. Hepatology 2014;60(2):715–35.
70. Gheorghe L, Iacob R, Vădan R, et al. Improvement of hepatic encephalopathy using a modified high-calorie high-protein diet. Rom J Gastroenterol 2005; 14(3):231–8.
71. Koretz R, Avenell A, Lipman T. Nutritional support for liver disease. Cochrane Database Syst Rev 2012;(5):CD008344.
72. Bunout D, Aicardi V, Hirsch S, et al. Nutritional support in hospitalized patients with alcoholic liver disease. Eur J Clin Nutr 1989;43(9):615–21.
73. Hayashi S, Aoyagi Y, Fujiwara K, et al. A randomized controlled trial of branched-chain amino acid (BCAA)-enriched elemental diet (ED-H) for hepatic encephalopathy [abstract]. J Gastroenterol Hepatol 1991;6(2):191.
74. Merli M, Riggio O. Dietary and nutritional indications in hepatic encephalopathy. Metab Brain Dis 2009;24(1):211–21.
75. Dam G, Ott P, Aagaard NK, et al. Branched-chain amino acids and muscle ammonia detoxification in cirrhosis. Metab Brain Dis 2013;28(2):217–20.
76. Holecek M. Branched-chain amino acids and ammonia metabolism in liver disease: therapeutic implications. Nutrition 2013;29(10):1186–91.
77. Muto Y, Sato S, Watanabe A, et al. Effects of oral branched-chain amino acid granules on event-free survival in patients with liver cirrhosis. Clin Gastroenterol Hepatol 2005;3:705–13.
78. Marchesini G, Bianchi G, Merli M, et al. Nutritional supplementation with branched-chain amino acids in advanced cirrhosis: a double-blind, randomized trial. Gastroenterology 2003;124(7):1792–801.
79. Gluud L, Dam G, Borre M, et al. Oral branched-chain amino acids have a beneficial effect on manifestations of hepatic encephalopathy in a systematic review with meta-analyses of randomized controlled trials. J Nutr 2013;143: 1263–8.
80. Rockey DC, Vierling JM, Mantry P, et al. Randomized, double-blind, controlled study of glycerol phenylbutyrate in hepatic encephalopathy. Hepatology 2014; 59(3):1073–83.
81. Kircheis G, Nilius R, Held C, et al. Therapeutic efficacy of l-ornithine-l-aspartate infusions in patients with cirrhosis and hepatic encephalopathy: results of a placebo-controlled, double-blind study. Hepatology 1997;25(6):1351–60.
82. Kristiansen RG, Rose CF, Fuskevåg O-M, et al. L-Ornithine phenylacetate reduces ammonia in pigs with acute liver failure through phenylacetylglycine formation: a novel ammonia-lowering pathway. Am J Physiol Gastrointest Liver Physiol 2014;307(10):G1024–31.
83. Ytrebø LM, Kristiansen RG, Maehre H, et al. L-ornithine phenylacetate attenuates increased arterial and extracellular brain ammonia and prevents intracranial hypertension in pigs with acute liver failure. Hepatology 2009;50(1):165–74.
84. Ventura-Cots M, Arranz J, Simón-Talero M, et al. Safety of ornithine phenylacetate in cirrhotic decompensated patients: an open-label, dose-escalating, single-cohort study. J Clin Gastroenterol 2013;47(10):881–7.
85. García PS, Cabbabe A, Kambadur R, et al. Brief-reports: elevated myostatin levels in patients with liver disease: a potential contributor to skeletal muscle wasting. Anesth Analg 2010;111(3):707–9.
86. Dasarathy S, McCullough AJ, Muc S, et al. Sarcopenia associated with portosystemic shunting is reversed by follistatin. J Hepatol 2011;54(5):915–21.

87. Plauth M, Schütz T, Buckendahl DP, et al. Weight gain after transjugular intrahepatic portosystemic shunt is associated with improvement in body composition in malnourished patients with cirrhosis and hypermetabolism. J Hepatol 2004;40(2): 228–33.
88. Tsien C, Shah SN, McCullough AJ, et al. Reversal of sarcopenia predicts survival after a transjugular intrahepatic portosystemic stent. Eur J Gastroenterol Hepatol 2013;25(1):85–93.
89. Román E, Torrades MT, Nadal MJ, et al. Randomized pilot study: effects of an exercise programme and leucine supplementation in patients with cirrhosis. Dig Dis Sci 2014;59(8):1966–75.

Ammonia and Its Role in the Pathogenesis of Hepatic Encephalopathy

 CrossMark

Parth J. Parekh, MD, Luis A. Balart, MD, MACG*

KEYWORDS

- Ammonia • Urea cycle • Hepatic encephalopathy • Astrocyte swelling • Glutamine
- Glutamate • GABA

KEY POINTS

- Hepatic encephalopathy (HE) is a commonly encountered sequela of chronic liver disease and cirrhosis with significant associated morbidity and mortality.
- Although ammonia is implicated in the pathogenesis of HE, the exact underlying mechanisms still remain poorly understood.
- Its role in the urea cycle, astrocyte swelling, and glutamine and gamma-amino-*n*-butyric acid systems suggests that the pathogenesis is multifaceted.
- Greater understanding of its underlying mechanism may offer more targeted therapeutic options in the future, and thus further research is necessary to fully understand the pathogenesis of HE.

INTRODUCTION

Hepatic encephalopathy (HE) or portosystemic encephalopathy is a sequela of chronic liver disease and cirrhosis with significant associated morbidity and mortality. A recent study found the annual inpatient incidence of HE to be 22,931, which is 0.33% of all hospitalizations in the United States, with an associated mortality of approximately 15%.[1] The inpatient cost burden of HE continues to increase, with the average inpatient cost in 2005 being $46,633 and in 2009 being $63,108 per hospitalization. Although the underlying mechanism remains poorly understood, the pathogenesis of HE is based on the accumulation of neurotoxins that are typically eliminated by the liver, including ammonia. This article provides an in-depth review of the role of ammonia in the pathogenesis of HE.

Disclosure: The authors have nothing to disclose.
Division of Gastroenterology and Hepatology, Department of Internal Medicine, Tulane University, New Orleans, LA, USA
* Corresponding author. Division of Gastroenterology and Hepatology, Tulane University, 1430 Tulane Avenue, New Orleans, LA 70112.
E-mail address: Lbalart@tulane.edu

Clin Liver Dis 19 (2015) 529–537
http://dx.doi.org/10.1016/j.cld.2015.05.002
1089-3261/15/$ – see front matter © 2015 Elsevier Inc. All rights reserved.

liver.theclinics.com

AMMONIA, THE UREA CYCLE, AND THE PATHOGENESIS OF HEPATIC ENCEPHALOPATHY

Ammonia is the best-characterized neurotoxin implicated in the pathogenesis of HE. Enterocytes[2] and colonic microflora[3] are thought to play a significant role in the production of ammonia from glutamine and the catabolism of nitrogenous sources in the form of ingested protein and secreted urea. In addition, recent studies have suggested that there may be an association with *Helicobacter pylori* (detected via biopsy of the gastric antrum or by ^{14}C urea breath test) and the pathogenesis of HE; however, its exact role remains unclear.[4–7]

In healthy individuals, the nitrogenous compounds generated by the gut microflora are transported to the liver via the portal circulation. In the liver, most of the nitrogenous compounds, along with endogenous nitrogen production via enterocytes and glutamine, enter the urea cycle to form urea and subsequently undergo renal excretion, as depicted in **Fig. 1**. **Fig. 2** depicts the difference in ammonia homeostasis in a healthy person versus one with cirrhosis.

In the case of advanced liver disease or cirrhosis, nitrogenous waste products (ie, ammonia) accumulate in the systemic circulation (hence the term portosystemic encephalopathy) because of damaged or nonfunctional hepatocytes and the development of portosystemic shunts, be they medically constructed or spontaneous, which bypass the liver.[8] Able to cross the blood-brain barrier, excess ammonia is then absorbed and metabolized by astrocytes and used to synthesize glutamine from glutamate via the enzyme glutamine synthetase.[9] The increased levels of glutamine create an osmotic gradient, resulting in increased osmotic pressure in the astrocytes causing morphologic changes similar to those of type II Alzheimer disease

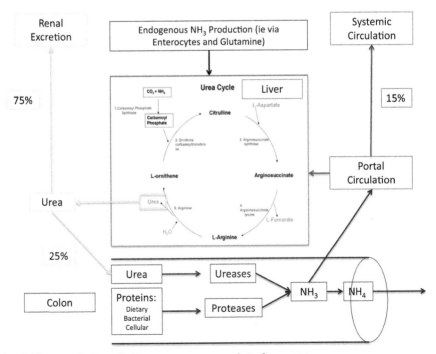

Fig. 1. The metabolism of nitrogenous compounds to form urea.

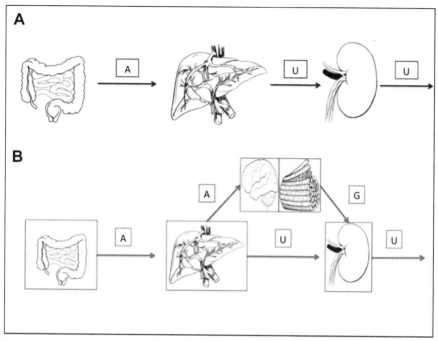

Fig. 2. Ammonia homeostasis. (*A*) Healthy. (*B*) Cirrhosis. A, ammonia; G, glutamine; U, urea.

characterized by cell swelling.[10–13] The net downstream effect is that of cerebral edema, increased intracranial pressure, and in severe cases brain herniation. Simultaneously occurring is an increase in activity of the gamma-amino-*n*-butyric acid (GABA) system resulting in a decrease of energy delivery to other neural cells and the subsequent production of endogenous benzodiazepines.[14,15]

AMMONIA AND ASTROCYTE SWELLING

As previously described, astrocytes use ammonia to form glutamine. Intracellular accumulation of glutamine results in astrocyte swelling, which ultimately results in neuronal dysfunction. Astrocyte swelling induces oxidative stress and forms reactive oxygen species, which further precipitates astrocyte swelling.[16] Görg and colleagues[17] sought to evaluate the role of oxidative/nitrosative stress in the pathogenesis of cerebral hyperammonemia. Postmortem cortical brain tissue samples from patients with cirrhosis with or without HE were compared with cortical brain tissue samples from patients without liver disease. In the cerebral cortices of the HE subgroup, there was noted to be significantly increased levels of tyrosine-nitrated proteins, heat shock protein-27, and 8-hydroxyguanosine, which are markers for RNA oxidation, suggesting a role of oxidative stress in the pathogenesis of HE.

Recent data have suggested that cognitive impairment may not resolve after an attack of overt HE, which is thought to be secondary to neuronal cells, namely astrocytes, entering a senescent state. Görg and colleagues[18] recently analyzed expression levels of senescence biomarkers in ammonia-treated rat astrocytes and in postmortem cortical brain tissue samples from cirrhotic patients with or without HE. Astrocyte proliferation was inhibited by ammonia, which was mediated by oxidative stress and activation of cell cycle inhibitory genes. In addition, mitochondria and the nucleus were identified as sources of radical oxygen species formation after prolonged exposure. The postmortem cortical tissues in patients with HE were found to have increased mRNA expression of senescence-associated genes, which were not found in those patients without HE. These data suggest that ammonia toxicity and HE are associated with astrocyte senescence, which ultimately impairs neurotransmission and contributes to cognitive impairment after an attack of overt HE. Recent clinical investigations evaluating the residual cognitive function of cirrhotic patients following clinical resolution of overt HE has shown persistent and cumulative deficits in working memory, response inhibition, and learning capacity.[19–21]

Lockwood and colleagues[22] postulated that cirrhotic patients with chronic exposure to increased ammonia levels adapt by increasing permeability surface area (PSA). Cerebral ammonia metabolism was studied in 5 control subjects and 5 patients with liver disease who were found to have minimal HE. The arterial ammonia concentration in the control subjects was 30 ± 7 µmol/L and 55 ± 13 µmol/L in patients with minimal HE. The cerebral blood flow, cerebral rate for ammonia, and the PSA product for ammonia were 0.58 ± 0.12 g^{-1} min^{-1}, 0.35 ± 0.15 µmol 100 g^{-1} min^{-1}, and 0.13 ± 0.3 mL g^{-1} min^{-1} in normal subjects respectively, compared with 0.46 ± 0.16 g^{-1} min^{-1}, 0.91 ± 0.36 µmol 100 g^{-1} min^{-1} ($P<.025$), and 0.22 ± 0.07 mL g^{-1} min^{-1} ($P>.05$) in patients with minimal HE, respectively. The increased PSA allows ammonia to diffuse across the blood-brain barrier more freely than normal and may explain the emergence of hypersensitivity with progression of liver disease despite normal or near-normal arterial ammonia levels.

Astrocyte swelling may occur independently of hyperammonemia. Other factors, such as benzodiazepines, hyponatremia, and inflammatory cytokines, have shown the ability to promote astrocyte swelling in vitro, which may also explain the presence of HE in patients with normal arterial ammonia levels.[10,11,23–25]

AMMONIA AND GLUTAMINE

On crossing the blood-brain barrier, ammonia acts as a necessary substrate in catalyzing glutamate to glutamine as a means of cerebral detoxification. Albrecht and Norenberg[26] questioned whether or not the synthesis of glutamine was benign, suggesting that it may be a noxious agent in and of itself via what they termed the 'Trojan Horse' model. These investigators suggest that newly synthesized glutamine is transported in excess (ie, the Trojan Horse) from the cytoplasm to mitochondria where it is metabolized by phosphate-activated glutaminase, resulting in the production of glutamate and ammonia. This glutamine-derived ammonia within the mitochondria results in mitochondrial dysfunction as it gives rise to reactive oxidative species and increasing mitochondrial permeability, itself resulting in astrocyte dysfunction and cell swelling.

Glutamine produced by astrocytes is an osmotically active molecule, which creates an osmotic gradient ultimately resulting in cerebral edema. Poveda and colleagues[27] investigated the dynamics of brain water in patients with cirrhosis and overt HE through MRI. Twenty-four patients with cirrhosis and overt HE were compared with 9 healthy controls and 9 controls with cirrhosis but without overt HE. Each patient underwent MRI and H-magnetic resonance spectroscopy in the first 24 hours after diagnosis of HE, and 5 were studied again 5 days after resolution of HE. A calculated glutamine/glutamate index was noted to be increased in HE compared with cirrhotic patients and healthy controls at 4.4, 2.4, and 1.8, respectively ($P = .0001$). Patients with overt HE revealed a decrease in magnetization transfer ratio values in several brain locations that did not resolve in those imaged 5 days after resolution of HE. The investigators concluded that cirrhotic patients with overt HE have a disturbance in osmolyte homeostasis causing low-grade edema that persists despite resolution of HE.

Recently, Sobczyk and colleagues[28] sought to evaluate the effect of ammonia on ephrine receptors (EphR) and their ligands (ephrines), because they are involved in the regulation of glutamate uptake by astrocytes and gliotransmitter release, thereby mitigating neurotransmission. Ammonium chloride was induced into messenger RNA (mRNA) and changes in EphR/ephrine isoforms measured in cultured astrocytes. There was a significant upregulation in EphR A4 mRNA in ammonium chloride–treated astrocytes, which was also noted in postmortem brain samples of cirrhotic patients with or without HE compared with controls. This finding suggests that ammonia modulates EphR/ephrine signaling in astrocytes.

AMMONIA AND GAMMA-AMINO-*N*-BUTYRIC ACID

Several studies have described the relationship between hyperammonemia and the increased inhibitory function of GABA as well as upregulation of 18-kDa translocator protein (TPSO).[29–32] Activation of TPSO is thought to result in the de novo production of endogenous benzodiazepines,[32] which in turn have modulatory properties on the GABA-A receptor that could potentially account for neuronal inhibition in HE.[33,34] There have been several proposed theories surrounding this relationship, with one theory focusing on tricarboxylic acid. Leke and colleagues[35] showed that ammonia induced increased tricarboxylic acid cycle activity and subsequently showed an increase in GABA synthesis via an indirect pathway in bile duct–ligated rats subjected to increased ammonia levels.[36] This premise has led to several studies using flumazenil in HE to reverse the effects of the endogenous benzodiazepines. A recent meta-analysis reviewed 6 double-blind randomized controlled trials, totaling 641 patients.[37] Approximately half the patients were treated with flumazenil and the other half with placebo. The mean percentage of patients showing clinical improvement was 27% in treated groups and 3% in patients who received placebo. In addition, there was modest electroencephalographic improvement in patients receiving flumazenil compared with placebo at 19% and 2%, respectively, suggesting that flumazenil may be beneficial in patients with HE.

There has been a recent paradigm shift focusing on TGR5 (Gpbar-1), a membrane-bound bile acid receptor with pleiotropic actions, which is expressed in astrocytes and neurons.[38] Keitel and colleagues[38] sought to establish its role as a neurosteroid receptor and found that stimulation in astrocytes results in the generation of reactive

Table 1
Classification of HE

Type	Underlying Cause	Subcategory	Subdivision
A	Acute liver failure	—	—
B	Portal-systemic shunting without associated intrinsic liver disease	—	—
C	Underlying cirrhosis and portal hypertension or portal-systemic shunts	Minimal	—
		Episodic	a. Precipitated
			b. Spontaneous
			c. Recurrent
		Persistent	a. Mild
			b. Severe
			c. Treatment dependent

Table 2 West-Haven criteria			
Stage	Level of Consciousness	Physical Examination Findings	Neurologic Examination Findings
0	Normal	Normal	Normal; psychomotor testing may indicate minimal HE[a]
1	Lack of awareness	Euphoria or anxiety; shortened attention span	Impaired performance of addition or subtraction; mild asterixis or tremor
2	Lethargic or apathetic	Minimal disorientation for time or place; subtle personality change; inappropriate behavior	Obvious asterixis; slurred speech
3	Somnolence to semistupor	Gross orientation; confusion; bizarre behavior	Clonus; muscle rigidity hyperreflexia
4	Coma	Coma (unresponsive to verbal or noxious stimuli)	Decerebrate posturing

[a] Shown to impair quality of life and increase risk of motor vehicle accidents.

oxygen species. In a rat model, the presence of ammonia downregulated TGR5 mRNA, which also coincided with downregulation seen in cerebral tissue sampled from cirrhotic patients with HE compared with noncirrhotic control subjects. This finding suggests that TGR5 may play a role in HE; however, its involvement remains to be fully studied.

CLASSIFICATION AND CLINICAL SUBTYPES
Classification

The World Congress of Gastroenterology first introduced a classification system in 1998, which subdivides HE depending on its underlying cause.[39] Type A describes HE associated with acute liver failure. Type B describes HE associated with portal-systemic shunting without associated intrinsic liver disease. Type C describes HE associated with underlying cirrhosis and portal hypertension or portal-systemic shunts. Type C is further subcategorized as minimal, episodic, or persistent. **Table 1** lists the classifications of HE.

Clinical Subtypes

The West-Haven Criteria is the most used classification system for grading severity of HE based on clinical presentation.[40] **Table 2** lists the West-Haven Criteria and associated physical examination and neurologic findings.

SUMMARY

HE is a commonly encountered sequela of chronic liver disease and cirrhosis with significant associated morbidity and mortality. Although ammonia is implicated in the pathogenesis of HE, the exact underlying mechanisms still remain poorly understood. Its role in the urea cycle, astrocyte swelling, and glutamine and GABA systems suggests that the pathogenesis is multifaceted. Greater understanding in its underlying mechanism may offer more targeted therapeutic options in the future, and thus further research is necessary to fully understand the pathogenesis of HE.

REFERENCES

1. Stepanova M, Mishra A, Venkatesan C, et al. In-hospital mortality and economic burden associated with hepatic encephalopathy in the United States from 2005 to 2009. Clin Gastroenterol Hepatol 2012;10(9):1034–41.e1.
2. Wu G, Knabe DA, Yan W, et al. Glutamine and glucose metabolism in enterocytes of the neonatal pig. Am J Physiol 1995;268(2 Pt 2):R334–42.
3. Richardson AJ, Mckain N, Wallace RJ. Ammonia production by human faecal bacteria, and the enumeration, isolation and characterization of bacteria capable of growth on peptides and amino acids. BMC Microbiol 2013;13:6.
4. Schulz C, Schütte K, Malfertheiner P, et al. Does *H. pylori* eradication therapy benefit patients with hepatic encephalopathy?: systematic review. J Clin Gastroenterol 2014;48(6):491–9.
5. Kountouras J, Zavos C, Deretzi G. *Helicobacter pylori* might contribute to persistent cognitive impairment after resolution of overt hepatic encephalopathy. Clin Gastroenterol Hepatol 2011;9(7):624.
6. Chen SJ, Wang LJ, Zhu Q, et al. Effect of *H pylori* infection and its eradication on hyperammonemia and hepatic encephalopathy in cirrhotic patients. World J Gastroenterol 2008;14(12):1914–8.
7. Zullo A, Hassan C, Morini S. Hepatic encephalopathy and *Helicobacter pylori*: a critical reappraisal. J Clin Gastroenterol 2003;37(2):164–8.
8. Poh Z, Chang PE. A current review of the diagnostic and treatment strategies of hepatic encephalopathy. Int J Hepatol 2012;2012:480309.
9. Brusilow SW. Hyperammonemic encephalopathy. Medicine (Baltimore) 2002; 81(3):240–9.
10. Häussinger D, Kircheis G, Fischer R, et al. Hepatic encephalopathy in chronic liver disease: a clinical manifestation of astrocyte swelling and low-grade cerebral edema? J Hepatol 2000;32(6):1035–8.
11. Häussinger D, Schliess F. Pathogenetic mechanisms of hepatic encephalopathy. Gut 2008;57(8):1156–65.
12. Miese F, Kircheis G, Wittsack HJ, et al. 1H-MR spectroscopy, magnetization transfer, and diffusion-weighted imaging in alcoholic and nonalcoholic patients with cirrhosis with hepatic encephalopathy. AJNR Am J Neuroradiol 2006;27(5): 1019–26.
13. Zhang XD, Zhang LJ, Wu SY, et al. Multimodality magnetic resonance imaging in hepatic encephalopathy: an update. World J Gastroenterol 2014;20(32): 11262–72.
14. Ahboucha S, Talani G, Fanutza T, et al. Reduced brain levels of DHEAS in hepatic coma patients: significance for increased GABAergic tone in hepatic encephalopathy. Neurochem Int 2012;61(1):48–53.
15. Sergeeva OA. GABAergic transmission in hepatic encephalopathy. Arch Biochem Biophys 2013;536(2):122–30.
16. Reinehr R, Görg B, Becker S, et al. Hypoosmotic swelling and ammonia increase oxidative stress by NADPH oxidase in cultured astrocytes and vital brain slices. Glia 2007;55(7):758–71.
17. Görg B, Qvartskhava N, Bidmon HJ, et al. Oxidative stress markers in the brain of patients with cirrhosis and hepatic encephalopathy. Hepatology 2010;52(1): 256–65.
18. Görg B, Karababa A, Shafigullina A, et al. Ammonia-induced senescence in cultured rat astrocytes and in human cerebral cortex in hepatic encephalopathy. Glia 2015;63(1):37–50.

19. Riggio O, Ridola L, Pasquale C, et al. Evidence of persistent cognitive impairment after resolution of overt hepatic encephalopathy. Clin Gastroenterol Hepatol 2011; 9(2):181–3.

20. Bajaj JS, Schubert CM, Heuman DM, et al. Persistence of cognitive impairment after resolution of overt hepatic encephalopathy. Gastroenterology 2010;138(7): 2332–40.

21. Umapathy S, Dhiman RK, Grover S, et al. Persistence of cognitive impairment after resolution of overt hepatic encephalopathy. Am J Gastroenterol 2014;109(7): 1011–9.

22. Lockwood AH, Yap EW, Wong WH. Cerebral ammonia metabolism in patients with severe liver disease and minimal hepatic encephalopathy. J Cereb Blood Flow Metab 1991;11(2):337–41.

23. Guevara M, Baccaro ME, Torre A, et al. Hyponatremia is a risk factor of hepatic encephalopathy in patients with cirrhosis: a prospective study with time-dependent analysis. Am J Gastroenterol 2009;104(6):1382–9.

24. Dasarathy S, Mullen KD. Benzodiazepines in hepatic encephalopathy: sleeping with the enemy. Gut 1998;42(6):764–5.

25. Seyan AS, Hughes RD, Shawcross DL. Changing face of hepatic encephalopathy: role of inflammation and oxidative stress. World J Gastroenterol 2010;16(27): 3347–57.

26. Albrecht J, Norenberg MD. Glutamine: a Trojan horse in ammonia neurotoxicity. Hepatology 2006;44(4):788–94.

27. Poveda MJ, Bernabeu A, Concepción L, et al. Brain edema dynamics in patients with overt hepatic encephalopathy: A magnetic resonance imaging study. Neuroimage 2010;52(2):481–7.

28. Sobczyk K, Jördens MS, Karababa A, et al. Ephrin/Ephrin receptor expression in ammonia-treated rat astrocytes and in human cerebral cortex in hepatic encephalopathy. Neurochem Res 2015;40(2):274–83.

29. Panickar KS, Jayakumar AR, Rama Rao KV, et al. Downregulation of the 18-kDa translocator protein: effects on the ammonia-induced mitochondrial permeability transition and cell swelling in cultured astrocytes. Glia 2007;55(16): 1720–7.

30. Ahboucha S, Butterworth RF. Pathophysiology of hepatic encephalopathy: a new look at GABA from the molecular standpoint. Metab Brain Dis 2004;19(3–4): 331–43.

31. Jones EA. Ammonia, the GABA neurotransmitter system, and hepatic encephalopathy. Metab Brain Dis 2002;17(4):275–81.

32. Ahboucha S, Gamrani H, Baker G. GABAergic neurosteroids: the "endogenous benzodiazepines" of acute liver failure. Neurochem Int 2012;60(7):707–14.

33. Butterworth RF. The astrocytic ("peripheral-type") benzodiazepine receptor: role in the pathogenesis of portal-systemic encephalopathy. Neurochem Int 2000; 36(4–5):411–6.

34. Ahboucha S. Neurosteroids and hepatic encephalopathy: an update on possible pathophysiologic mechanisms. Curr Mol Pharmacol 2011;4(1):1–13.

35. Leke R, Bak LK, Schousboe A, et al. Demonstration of neuron-glia transfer of precursors for GABA biosynthesis in a co-culture system of dissociated mouse cerebral cortex. Neurochem Res 2008;33(12):2629–35.

36. Leke R, Bak LK, Iversen P, et al. Synthesis of neurotransmitter GABA via the neuronal tricarboxylic acid cycle is elevated in rats with liver cirrhosis consistent with a high GABAergic tone in chronic hepatic encephalopathy. J Neurochem 2011;117(5):824–32.

37. Goulenok C, Bernard B, Cadranel JF, et al. Flumazenil vs. placebo in hepatic encephalopathy in patients with cirrhosis: a meta-analysis. Aliment Pharmacol Ther 2002;16(3):361–72.
38. Keitel V, Görg B, Bidmon HJ, et al. The bile acid receptor TGR5 (Gpbar-1) acts as a neurosteroid receptor in brain. Glia 2010;58(15):1794–805.
39. Ferenci P, Lockwood A, Mullen K, et al. Hepatic encephalopathy–definition, nomenclature, diagnosis, and quantification: final report of the working party at the 11th World Congresses of Gastroenterology, Vienna, 1998. Hepatology 2002;35(3):716–21.
40. Gundling F, Zelihic E, Seidl H, et al. How to diagnose hepatic encephalopathy in the emergency department. Ann Hepatol 2013;12(1):108–14.

Novel Ammonia-Lowering Agents for Hepatic Encephalopathy

Robert S. Rahimi, MD, MS[a],*, Don C. Rockey, MD[b]

KEYWORDS

- AST-120 • Cirrhosis • Glycerol phenylbutyrate • MARS • Ornithine phenylacetate
- Benzoate • Polyethylene glycol • PEG

KEY POINTS

- Glycerol phenylbutyrate (GPB) decreases the likelihood of being hospitalized for hepatic encephalopathy (HE) or experiencing an overall hepatic encephalopathy event compared with placebo.
- Ornithine phenylacetate (OP) enhances the excretion of ammonia in the urine as phenylacetylglutamine (PAGN); a phase IIb trial is currently investigating its use for acute HE.
- Polyethylene glycol (PEG) seems an effective alternative to treat acute HE (compared with lactulose), with a potential to decrease hospital length of stay.

INTRODUCTION

Hepatic encephalopathy (HE) is a common and devastating complication of cirrhosis. The spectrum of HE ranges from covert HE (previously termed minimal HE) to overt HE (previously termed acute HE) and accounts for frequent hospitalization, decrease in the quality of life, and poorer outcomes than in cirrhotic patients who have not had HE.

Although it is long been believed that ammonia produced by gut bacteria is an important contributing factor to the pathogenesis of HE, HE is a multifactorial disease (**Fig. 1**) process for which the underlying mechanisms leading to altered cerebral function are still not well understood.[1] The production of ammonia can arise from gram-negative anaerobes (ie, *Enterobacteriaceae*, *Proteus*, and *Clostridium* species) that have bacterial urease, converting urea from the blood into ammonia and carbon dioxide.[2–4] One of the purported mechanisms of action for lactulose is that it helps clear

Dr R.S. Rahimi receives research support from Ocera Therapeutics, and Dr D.C. Rockey receives research support from the NIH, Hyperion Therapeutics, and Gilead Sciences.
^a Annette C. and Harold C. Simmons Transplant Institute, Baylor University Medical Center, 3410 Worth Street, Suite 860, Dallas, TX 75246, USA; ^b Department of Internal Medicine, Medical University of South Carolina, 96 Jonathan Lucas Street, Room 803 CSB, Charleston, SC 29425, USA
* Corresponding author.
E-mail address: robert.rahimi@baylorhealth.edu

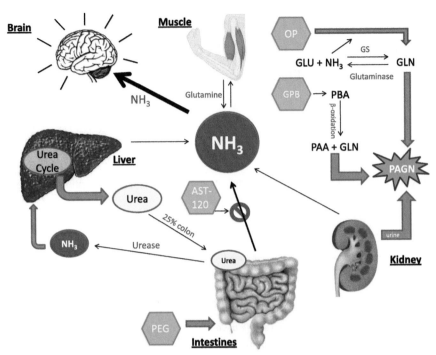

Fig. 1. Multiorgan ammonia (NH₃) pathways with specific NH₃-lowering medications used in cirrhosis. Circulating concentrations of NH₃ are shown with multiorgan involvement in the production of NH₃, ultimately resulting in NH₃ crossing the blood-brain barrier, contributing to astrocyte swelling and HE, because decreased urea cycle capability and reduced liver glutamine synthetase (GS) activity is present in cirrhosis. The alternative pathway is shown at the top, where NH₃ binds with glutamate (GLU)-forming glutamine (GLN) after enzymatic processing using GS. Both ornithine phenylacetate (OP) and glycerol phenylbutyrate (GPB) are NH₃-lowering medications; they combine GLN and phenylacetate (PAA) to form phenyl-acetylglutamine (PAGN), which is excreted in the urine. AST-120 is a carbon microsphere adsorbent, which binds NH₃ in the gut, thus lowering circulating NH₃ levels. Polyethylene glycol (PEG) is a cathartic, which causes rapid clearance of gut bacterial synthesizing NH₃ to be excreted into the feces. Approximately one-fourth of urea-derived byproducts from the urea cycle is shunted to the colon (not shown; remaining three-fourths of urea excreted in the kidneys), where urease-producing bacterial organisms produce NH₃ that enters the portal circulation. Skeletal muscle also contributes in the regulation of NH₃, as depicted. Not shown is the presence of GS and glutaminase in each organ, contributing to NH₃ homeostasis. PBA, phenylbutyric acid. NH3 circles represent circulating ammonia.

the GI tract of ammonia producing bacteria. Additionally, enterocytes in the small bowel seem to generate ammonia via intestinal glutaminase, an enzyme that metabolizes glutamine into glutamate and ammonia[5,6] and is found up-regulated in cirrhotic patients with minimal and overt HE.[7,8] Additionally, because the ability of the liver to clear ammonia is diminished in cirrhosis, and because portal hypertension leads to shunting of blood around the sinusoids, cirrhosis leads to hyperammonemia. The ensuing elevation in ammonia is thought to cause oxidative dysfunction in the mitochondria of astrocytes, resulting in cerebral edema and neurologic dysfunction.[9] Regardless of the precise mechanism of hyperammonemia, because it is thought to be a major underlying mechanism contributing to the development of HE, this review focuses on novel ammonia-lowering approaches in HE.

AMMONIA SCAVENGERS

Ammonia scavengers that are approved for use in patients with urea cycle disorders and hyperammonemia, mostly in children, include sodium benzoate (combines with glycine) and sodium phenylacetate (combines with glutamine)—distributed under the trade name Ammonul (Ucyclyd Pharma, Inc., Scottsdale, AZ)—to form water-soluble, renally excretable compounds (benzoylglycine or hippurate and PAGN, respectively) that eliminate ammonia through the urine (see **Fig. 1**; **Table 1**). Oral sodium benzoate (Ucyclyd Pharma, Inc., Scottsdale, AZ) is also sometimes used off-label for ammonia scavenging and is available in powder form from specialty pharmacies. Although these products are available in the United States, they are not approved for HE. A critical consideration with their use is the need to use a large therapeutic dose (measured in grams per day), which leads to a significant sodium load (1–2 g/d at therapeutic doses). This is problematic for several reasons, including that they may contribute to fluid retention in cirrhotic patients and may also lead to hypernatremia, which in turn may cause an alteration in mental status. Additionally, these compounds taste salty and are thus are difficult for patients to take. GPB (HPN-100, Hyperion Therapeutics, South San Francisco, California) improves the organoleptic properties of its predecessor, a prodrug of phenylacetate (PAA), oral sodium phenylbutyrate (Buphenyl [Sigmapharm Laboratories, LLC., Bensalem, PA]); it avoids the risk of sodium overload and has been shown safe and well tolerated.[10,11]

Glycerol Phenylbutyrate

GPB is a nearly tasteless, odorless, sodium-free liquid compound that is a prodrug of sodium phenylbutyrate, whose mechanism of action is removal of nitrogen excretion

Table 1
Clinical features and approved uses for the different types of medicines that act as ammonia scavengers

Ammonia Scavengers	Appearance	Mechanism of Action/Byproduct	Dosage	Approved Use
Sodium benzoate	White or colorless crystalline powder	1 mol of Nitrogen removed/mole of benzoate after conjugated with glycine	5.5 g/m² IV over 90–120 min, repeat daily	Urea cycle disorders Food preservative
Sodium phenylacetate	White to off-white crystalline powder	2 mol of Nitrogen removed/mole of PAA after conjugated with glutamine		Urea cycle disorders
GPB	Colorless to pale yellow liquid	Nitrogen removal in the form of urinary PAGN	5–12.4 g/m² daily	Urea cycle disorders
OP	Crystalline salt	Nitrogen removal in the form of urinary PAGN	10 g IV daily	Possibly future approval for overt HE
AST-120	Charcoal powder	Binding of neuroactive substances (including ammonia) in the GI tract	6–12 g IV daily	Delaying dialysis in chronic kidney disease; uremic symptoms

in the form of urinary PAGN, allowing an alternative pathway for ammonia waste (**Fig. 2**).[12] It has been approved for inherited disorders causing hyperammonemia, including treatment of urea cycle deficiencies.[13–16]

Because GPB has been shown to lower ammonia, an open-label pilot study assessed the tolerability and effect on venous ammonia in cirrhotic patients with HE in 15 patients given 6 mL versus 9 mL of GPB orally twice daily with food for 4 weeks.[10] Fasting ammonia concentrations were lower on GPB compared with baseline, with a decrease in ammonia levels to 45.4 (27.9) μmol/L (upper limit of normal approximately 48 μmol/L), on the eighth day of 6 mL, twice-a-day GPB dosing, $P<.05$); 9 mL twice a day yielded similar lowering but was associated with more adverse events and higher PAA plasma concentrations.

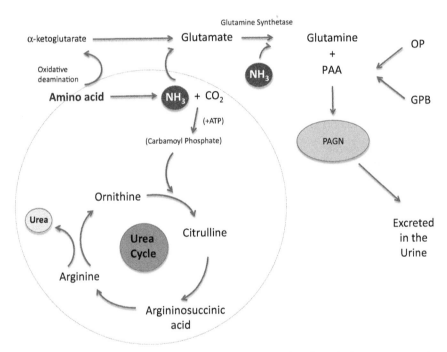

Fig. 2. Ammonia (NH_3) metabolism by the urea (ornithine) cycle and alternate ammonium excretion pathways. NH_3 is the product of oxidative deamination reactions and is an end product of amino acid/protein metabolism. Thus, NH_3 is a waste product, which is normally converted to urea and excreted in the urea cycle, as depicted within the circle. The addition of NH_3 to the urea cycle results in urea and ornithine formation. In patients with liver disease and hepatocellular dysfunction, enzymatic processes in dysfunctional hepatocytes are presumably unable to handle NH_3, resulting in accumulation of NH_3. In the upper portion of the figure, an alternative pathway exists in which glutamine synthetase uses NH_3 and glutamate as substrates to form glutamine. Glutamine then combines with PAA (the active moiety in sodium phenylbutyrate after conjugation of glutamine in the liver) to form PAGN. Ornithine phenylacetate (OP) (combines with ornithine and ammonia produced from skeletal muscle after glutamine synthesis) and glycerol phenylbutyrate (GPB) provide phenylacetate (PAA) as substrate (GPB is metabolized to phenylbutyric acid in the intestine and undergoes β-oxidation in the liver and other organs to form PAA). PAA and glutamine (by the action of glutamine N-acyltransferase) are combined to form phenylacetylglutamine (PAGN), which is harmlessly excreted into the urine; this alternative pathway allows NH_3 and excess nitrogen waste to be excreted from the body.

This study provided the impetus to perform a multicenter, randomized, double-blind, placebo-controlled phase II trial to test the hypothesis that ammonia lowering using GPB (6 mL twice a day for 16 weeks in patients with HE) would decrease the incidence of HE events in patients with cirrhosis and a history of at least 2 HE episodes of greater than or equal to grade 2 within the past 6 months, including 1 event within 3 months of randomization (Clinicaltrials.gov, NCT00999167).[11] Patients were excluded for the following reasons: use of other ammonia-lowering agents (eg, L-ornithine-L-aspartate and sodium benzoate); active complications of cirrhosis (sepsis, hepatocellular carcinoma, hepatic hydrothorax, and so forth); gastrointestinal (GI) bleeding requiring blood transfusion within 3 months; transjugular intrahepatic portosystemic shunt placement or revision within 90 days; recreational drug use or alcohol consumption for patients with a history of alcohol or drug abuse within 6 months; regular use of benzodiazepines, narcotics, or barbiturates; prolonged QT interval; Model for End-Stage Liver Disease (MELD) score greater than 25; serum creatinine greater than 2 mg/dL, serum sodium less than 125 mEq/L; platelet count less than 35,000/μL; hemoglobin less than 8 g/dL; hematocrit less than 25%; expected liver transplantation within 6 months; and hypersensitivity to GPB or its metabolites. Patients taking rifaximin were eligible if they had experienced at least 1 of their 2 qualifying HE events after taking rifaximin for at least 1 month.

In this trial, 178 patients were enrolled and included in the intention-to-treat analysis; 61% (55/90) in the GPB arm versus 76% (67/88) in the placebo arm completed therapy, with 54% (19/35) in the GPB arm versus 76% (16/21) in the placebo arm meeting predetermined stopping rules. Baseline characteristics were similar between the 2 groups, including lactulose use; however, more Child-Pugh class C patients were randomized to GPB than to placebo (21 vs 8, respectively), and fewer men were randomized to GPB than to placebo (45 vs 59) with only US patients using rifaximin at baseline. In the intention-to-treat population, a lower proportion of patients in the GPB group compared with the placebo group experienced an HE event (21% vs 36%; $P = .02$), meeting the primary endpoint. Also time to first event (hazard ratio [HR] = 0.56; $P < .05$), total events (35 vs 57; $P = .04$), and fewer HE hospitalizations (13 vs 25; $P = .06$) occurred in the GPB versus placebo arms, respectively. Among patients not on rifaximin at enrollment, GPB had even more prominent effects, reducing the proportion of patients with an HE event (10% vs 32%; $P < .01$), time to first event (HR = 0.29; $P < .01$), and total events (7 vs 31; $P < .01$). Adverse events (nearly 75% in each group) were similar in both groups, and plasma ammonia was significantly lower in patients on GPB, which correlated with HE events when measured either at baseline or during the study.

These data indicate that GPB improved outcomes, decreased ammonia levels, and was considered safe among patients with cirrhosis with recurrent HE. The results suggest that GPB may be used to prevent HE in patients with recurrent HE. A further larger, randomized trial is anticipated to further establish the role of GPB in patients with HE.

Ornithine Phenylacetate

OP (OCR-002) combines ornithine and PAA in a crystalline salt and has been shown to decrease ammonia and enhance the disposal of nitrogenous molecules in urine by 2 mechanisms. First, L-ornithine acts as a substrate for glutamine synthesis from ammonia in skeletal muscle, and second, PAA enhances the excretion of the ornithine-related glutamine as PAGN in the kidney (see **Fig. 2**).[17] The safety and tolerability of OP in cirrhotic patients with upper GI bleeding was evaluated, exploring its effects on blood ammonia and plasma and urine metabolites during 5 days of continuous infusions.[18] The investigators enrolled 10 patients of 26 subjects with upper

GI bleeding who followed standard treatment protocols and matched them for Child-Pugh stage and plasma creatinine to patients who received OP. Exclusion criteria included the following: signs of HE, need for mechanical ventilation, terminal illness, infection by HIV, neurologic comorbidities that might impair mental status, suspected hypersensitivity or allergic reaction to the drug components, electrocardiogram with QT interval–corrected Fridericia greater than 500 ms (Bazett formula), creatinine greater than 1.5 mg/dL, and need for hemodialysis. Patients taking the following drugs were also excluded: penicillin, probenecid, haloperidol, valproic acid, and systemic corticosteroids. The initial OP dose was 0.138 g/h, and this was increased to 0.275 g/h after 12 hours and to 0.416 g/h after 24 hours, with incremental dose adjustments if patients did not develop predefined stopping criteria. All 10 patients completed the study with 5 continuous days of intravenous (IV) OP infusion, achieving a target dose of 10 g/d. The mean age was 60 years; 90% (9/10) were male; 70% (7/10) were Child-Pugh class A; B: 30% (3/10) were Child-Pugh class B; 60% (6/10) had Laennec cirrhosis; 20% (2/10) had hepatitis C; 10% (1/10) had hepatitis B; and 10% (1/10) had cryptogenic cirrhosis. Plasma ammonia was significantly higher in the control group at 24 hours and showed a progressive decline between baseline (80 $\pm$ 43 μmol/L), 36 hours (42 $\pm$ 15 μmol/L), 72 hours (44 $\pm$ 15 μmol/L), 96 hours (40 $\pm$ 24 μmol/L), and 120 hours (33 $\pm$ 14 μmol/L). Plasma glutamine also decreased (−37% at day 5), with its excretion in urine as PAGN progressively rising (52 $\pm$ 35 mmol at day 5). No serious adverse events were reported. Currently, OP is under clinical development in decompensated cirrhosis for overt HE, with phase IIb study results expected in 2016. This compound thus may prove useful for treating acute HE.[19]

Spherical Carbon Adsorbent (AST-120)

AST-120 (Ocera Therapeutics, San Diego, California) is an orally formulated carbon microsphere (0.2–0.4 mm in diameter) adsorbent, engineered with highly nonspecific surface area (>1600 m^2/g), that was approved in Japan in 1991 to improve uremia and delay the initiation of dialysis in patients with chronic renal insufficiency.[20–23] Although AST-120 differs structurally from activated charcoal, it exhibits superior adsorption for certain organic compounds (ie, low molecular weight <10 kDa) from the lumen of the lower GI tract due to its unique nanopore volume and size, allowing for a selective binding surface (see **Fig. 1**).[24] Because AST-120 is not degraded or adsorbed from the GI tract, minimal interference with digestive enzymes or drug absorption is seen, rendering it safe for prolonged use.

AST-120 has been shown to lower plasma ammonia levels in portacaval shunted dogs,[25] and preliminary studies in humans with low-grade HE have shown neurocognitive benefits after AST-120 therapy.[26] More recently, AST-120 has been shown to have ammonia-lowering capabilities, including binding of a variety of neuroactive substances linked to the pathogenesis of HE, thereby mitigating brain edema. AST-120 was shown to lower arterial ammonia, oxidative stress, brain edema, and locomotor activity in rats induced with secondary biliary cirrhosis after bile-duct ligation (BDL).[27] In vitro assessments of AST-120, using ranges of solutions reported in humans with HE,[28] demonstrated 60% adsorption of ammonia within the first hour, with 77% to 94% adsorption occurring after 6 hours of incubation at different concentrations. In vivo, AST-120 was administered to both BDL and sham control rats for either (1) 6 weeks by gavage every 12 hours at doses of 0.1, 1, and 4 g/kg/d, starting 1 day after surgery; (2) 3 days of 1 g/kg/d, starting 39 days after surgery; or (3) 2 weeks of 1 g/kg/d, starting 4 weeks after surgery. In the 6-week preventative group, arterial ammonia increased in nontreated BDL rats compared with sham controls (177.3 $\pm$ 30.8 μM vs 66.5 $\pm$ 18.2 μM; $P<.01$), whereas all doses of AST-120 decreased ammonia in a dose-dependent manner in BDL rats (121.9 ± 13.8 μM; 80.9 ± 30.0 μM; and 48.8 ± 19.6 μM) to levels found in sham controls (81.1 ± 8.9 μM; 72.2 ± 6.3 μM; and 53.8 ± 16.8 μM) using concentrations of 0.1, 1, and 4 g/kg/d, respectively. Ammonia levels correlated with the dose of AST-120 (Spearman ρ = −0.6603; P = .0006) and were significantly lower in treated BDL versus nontreated BDL rats (P<.01). Brain water content in the frontal cortex (79.39% ± 0.22% vs 78.60% ± 0.19%; P<.05), cerebellum (78.89% ± 0.16% vs 77.96% ± 0.16%; P<.01), and brain-stem (69.50% ± 0.25% vs 68.78% ± 0.41%; P<.01) was significantly increased in nontreated BDL rats versus nontreated sham controls. After therapy with AST-120, brain water content in all areas studied demonstrated similar values to their respective sham-operated controls. The effect of AST-120 on short-term treatment, administered for either 3 days or 2 weeks after surgery, significantly reduced arterial ammonia levels and brain water content in all 3 regions, in comparison with nontreated BDL animals, relative to sham-operated controls (P<.05). Locomotor activity in BDL rats was reduced compared with sham controls but normalized after AST-120 therapy; however, reactive oxygen species levels remained unchanged. Furthermore, AST-120 attenuated an increase in blood ammonia after IV-infused ammonium acetate was given, thereby preventing progression to precoma in BDL-treated rats in comparison to nontreated rats (P<.05).

A multicenter, double-blind, randomized, placebo-controlled trial was performed to evaluate the overall safety, tolerability, and effectiveness of AST-120 in 148 patients with compensated cirrhosis (with MELD scores less than 25) and covert HE; AST-120 was given for 8 weeks.[29] The mean age was 55 years, MELD score was 10, and 53% had chronic hepatitis C. Patients were randomized to receive AST-120, 12 g (n = 50); AST-120, 6 g (n = 50); or placebo (n = 48). There were no baseline differences in psychometric scores, clinical global assessment of HE, or overt HE/hospitalizations between all groups at baseline. Although venous ammonia decreased significantly from baseline after 8 weeks of treatment in both AST-120 groups compared with placebo, this was independent of neurocognitive improvement. The investigators suggested that AST-120 was well tolerated but did not meet the primary endpoint of improvement in the Repeatable Battery for the Assessment of Neuropsychological Status (RBANS) due to a confounding study design, allowing improvement in neurocognitive measures before randomization. The final phase II study results are awaited, to be reported in full form before final recommendations can be made; however, further investigation most likely will be needed.

Molecular Adsorbent Recirculating System and Bioartificial Devices

Extracorporeal devices that remove ammonia from the body are attractive therapeutic alternatives for patients with HE. Although several of these liver or albumin dialysis systems are currently available, the Molecular Adsorbent Recirculating System (MARS) (Baxter Intl., Deerfield, IL) represents the classic device, which was granted Food and Drug Administration approval in January 2013 for the treatment of HE, and is used in more than 45 countries worldwide, although mostly for research purposes because it is considered a costly procedure. These devices have been evaluated most commonly in patients with refractory HE, often in patients with acute liver failure. In patients with cirrhosis and refractory HE, the MARS was studied in a large, multicenter, randomized controlled trial for patients with severe HE and not responding to standard treatment.[30] The MARS, used for 6 hours daily for 5 days or until the patient had greater than or equal to 2 grade improvement in HE, was compared with standard medical therapy (SMT). The primary endpoint was to evaluate the difference in improvement of HE between the 2 groups. Of the 70 patients with a median age and MELD score of 53 years and 32, respectively, 44% were female, having severe HE (grade 3, 56%; grade 4, 44%). Patients were randomized to MARS plus SMT (n = 39) or SMT alone (n = 31), with higher improvement of HE in the MARS plus SMT group (mean, 34%) versus the SMT group (mean, 19%), $P = .044$, and was reached at a more frequent and rapid rate compared with the SMT group ($P = .045$). Overall MARS therapy was tolerated well with no unexpected adverse events; however, no benefit regarding mortality was demonstrated between the 2 groups.

Other devices, including bioartificial machines with hepatocytes, have been studied for treatment of HE.[31] In 1 study, 18 patients with grade 2 to 4 acute HE who did not respond to at least 24 hours of medical therapy received a maximum of three 6-hour charcoal based hemodiabsorption treatments. The mean time to improvement in HE grade less than or equal to 2 or at least a 50% HE index reduction was 2.6 ± 1.9 days, and 89% (16/18) of patients had a response. Survival was 94% and 72% at 5 and 30 days, respectively. This and other similar therapies, however, are not currently approved for use in the United States.

POLYETHYLENE GLYCOL

Because gut bacteria synthesize ammonia, it follows that their rapid clearance might result in a benefit in patients with HE. This has been the authors' clinical experience with the use of PEG. This led to a randomized clinical trial to study the effect of PEG in acute HE (Clinicaltrials.gov, NCT01283152) (see **Fig. 1**).[32] In this study, in which 186 cirrhotic patients admitted for overt HE were screened and 50 patients met inclusion criteria, of whom 25 patients received a 4-L dose of PEG and 25 patients received SMT with lactulose. The 2 groups were similar with respect to demographics, laboratory, and clinical features, with the exception of blood urea nitrogen (BUN), which was higher in the PEG group ($P = .03$); 78% of patients received 1 dose of lactulose per emergency department SMT protocol prior to randomization (lactulose arm, n = 19; PEG arm, n = 20), whereas the remaining 22% were recruited prior to lactulose administration. There were no significant differences among the groups with regard to the initial dosing with lactulose ($P = .45$). The primary outcome was improvement in at least 1 HE grade using the HE scoring algorithm (HESA) within 24 hours for both groups. Initial HESA scores were identical (mean 2.3, $P = .70$) and there were no differences in the distribution of the scores ($P = .62$). In the lactulose group, 36% (9 of 25 total subjects) had an incremental improvement of 1 HESA grade, 3 (12%) improved by 2 grades, and 1 (4%) improved by 3 HESA grades at 24 hours; 48% (12 of 25 subjects) had no improvement. Only 2 had a HESA score of zero (8%) at 24 hours. In contrast, 43% (10 of 23 subjects) improved by 1 HESA grade at 24 hours, 9 (39%) by 2 grades, and 1 by 3 grades (4%); 9% (2 of 23 subjects receiving PEG) had no improvement. Ten subjects (43%) had a HESA score of zero at 24 hours. Overall, subjects receiving PEG had a significantly lower mean HESA score at 24 hours than patients receiving lactulose ($0.9 ± 1.0$ vs $1.6 ± 0.9$; $P = .002$). The median time to HE resolution was 1 day in subjects receiving PEG compared with 2 days in receiving SMT lactulose ($P = .01$). Another important point is that hospital length of stay was reduced in patients receiving PEG ($4 ± 3$ days) compared with controls ($8 ± 12$ days; $P = .07$). There were no definitive adverse related events reported with either lactulose or PEG.

With regard to ammonia, excretion in the stool has been previously shown greater with PEG than with lactulose.[33] Thus, an interesting observation occurred in this study was that the 24-hour change in blood ammonia was greater in the lactulose group than in the PEG group; furthermore, ammonia levels did not correlate with better improvement in HESA grades (**Table 2**). Possible explanations for this result could be the

Table 2
Hepatic Encephalopathy: Lactulose vs Polyethylene Glycol 3350-Electrolyte Solution (HELP) study outcomes

Variable	Total	Lactulose	PEG	P Value[a]
24-h Change in HESA (mean ± SD)	1.1 ± 0.8	0.7 ± 0.8	1.5 ± 0.8[b]	.002
24-h Change in ammonia				
Elapsed time = 6–24 h	(n = 33)	(n = 15)	(n = 18)	—
Before-study prescription (μmol/L)	159 ± 73	175 ± 70	146 ± 75	.19
After-study prescription (μmol/L)	103 ± 51	82 ± 29	120 ± 60	.049
Difference in level (μmol/L)	56 ± 88	93 ± 71	26 ± 90	.025
Length of stay[b]	6 ± 9	8 ± 12	4 ± 3	.07

[a] Comparison of control (lactulose) and experimental (PEG) groups using Wilcoxon (Mann-Whitney) rank sum for ammonia and HESA, Kaplan-Meier for length of stay, and Fisher exact test for categorical variables.
[b] 24-Hour HESA on 2 patients: 1 was competent and refused testing and 1 was discharged in less than 24 hours; initial HESA was omitted from analysis.
From Rahimi RS, Singal AG, Cuthbert JA, et al. Lactulose vs polyethylene glycol 3350-electrolyte solution for treatment of overt hepatic encephalopathy: the HELP randomized clinical trial. JAMA Intern Med 2014;174:1730; with permission.

mechanism of action of the 2 study medications[33] and to the timing of the post-treatment ammonia level. Because PEG is a highly effective cathartic, the potential clinical improvement in HE might precede and be more clinically relevant than the actual decrease in ammonia levels, which parallels the authors' hypothesis in this study. Alternatively, circulating ammonia levels may return to their elevated baseline faster (and before clinical deterioration is manifested). PEG may also in theory result in dehydration and decreased renal perfusion, which might lead to decreased renal ammonia excretion. Future studies evaluating ammonia and its correlation with HE resolution will likely help clarify this issue.

Given the theoretic possibility that PEG treatment may lead to alterations in electrolyte levels or renal function, this was also assessed in this study. Electrolytes, creatinine, and BUN were measured at baseline and at 6 to 24 hours after admission. Potassium levels decreased from 4.3 mmol/L to 3.8 mmol/L after PEG ($P = .006$). Six subjects in each the PEG and lactulose groups had moderate hypokalemia (potassium <3.5 mmol/L) during the first 6 to 24 hours after treatment. There were no significant changes in serum sodium, creatinine, or BUN after either PEG or lactulose treatment.

The data suggest that bowel cleansing with PEG, normally used for colonoscopy preparations, is a safe, rapid, and effective immediate management strategy for subjects presenting with acute overt HE compared with the current SMT lactulose. Because the effect of PEG is transient, however, follow-up therapy with lactulose to prevent recurrence of HE in those with chronic symptoms is important.

SUMMARY

Many recent studies have provided insight in the management of patients with cirrhosis and HE, either acute (overt) or chronic (covert), with regard to newer pharmacologic agents that decrease ammonia levels. Ammonia scavengers, including GPB and OP, seem promising, whereas liver dialysis machines might have future use beyond the research spectrum. AST-120 and PEG have been implemented in acute HE; however, further research is still required.

REFERENCES

1. Blei AT, Cordoba J. Hepatic encephalopathy. Am J Gastroenterol 2001;96: 1968–76.
2. Vince AJ, Burridge SM. Ammonia production by intestinal bacteria: the effects of lactose, lactulose and glucose. J Med Microbiol 1980;13:177–91.
3. Floch MH, Katz J, Conn HO. Qualitative and quantitative relationships of the fecal flora in cirrhotic patients with portal systemic encephalopathy and following portacaval anastomosis. Gastroenterology 1970;59:70–5.
4. Wolpert E, Phillips SF, Summerskill WH. Ammonia production in the human colon. Effects of cleansing, neomycin and acetohydroxamic acid. N Engl J Med 1970; 283:159–64.
5. Plauth M, Roske AE, Romaniuk P, et al. Post-feeding hyperammonaemia in patients with transjugular intrahepatic portosystemic shunt and liver cirrhosis: role of small intestinal ammonia release and route of nutrient administration. Gut 2000;46:849–55.
6. Olde Damink SW, Jalan R, Redhead DN, et al. Interorgan ammonia and amino acid metabolism in metabolically stable patients with cirrhosis and a TIPSS. Hepatology 2002;36:1163–71.
7. Romero-Gomez M, Ramos-Guerrero R, Grande L, et al. Intestinal glutaminase activity is increased in liver cirrhosis and correlates with minimal hepatic encephalopathy. J Hepatol 2004;41:49–54.
8. Romero-Gomez M, Jover M, Del Campo JA, et al. Variations in the promoter region of the glutaminase gene and the development of hepatic encephalopathy in patients with cirrhosis: a cohort study. Ann Intern Med 2010;153:281–8.
9. Haussinger D, Kircheis G, Fischer R, et al. Hepatic encephalopathy in chronic liver disease: a clinical manifestation of astrocyte swelling and low-grade cerebral edema? J Hepatol 2000;32:1035–8.
10. Ghabril M, Zupanets IA, Vierling J, et al. Glycerol phenylbutyrate in patients with cirrhosis and episodic hepatic encephalopathy: a pilot study of safety and effect on venous ammonia concentration. Clin Pharm Drug Dev 2013;2:278–84.
11. Rockey DC, Vierling JM, Mantry P, et al. Randomized, double-blind, controlled study of glycerol phenylbutyrate in hepatic encephalopathy. Hepatology 2014; 59:1073–83.
12. Lee B, Rhead W, Diaz GA, et al. Phase 2 comparison of a novel ammonia scavenging agent with sodium phenylbutyrate in patients with urea cycle disorders: safety, pharmacokinetics and ammonia control. Mol Genet Metab 2010;100: 221–8.
13. McGuire BM, Zupanets IA, Lowe ME, et al. Pharmacology and safety of glycerol phenylbutyrate in healthy adults and adults with cirrhosis. Hepatology 2010;51: 2077–85.
14. Diaz GA, Krivitzky LS, Mokhtarani M, et al. Ammonia control and neurocognitive outcome among urea cycle disorder patients treated with glycerol phenylbutyrate. Hepatology 2013;57:2171–9.
15. Lichter-Konecki U, Diaz GA, Merritt JL 2nd, et al. Ammonia control in children with urea cycle disorders (UCDs); phase 2 comparison of sodium phenylbutyrate and glycerol phenylbutyrate. Mol Genet Metab 2011;103:323–9.
16. Smith W, Diaz GA, Lichter-Konecki U, et al. Ammonia control in children ages 2 months through 5 years with urea cycle disorders: comparison of sodium phenylbutyrate and glycerol phenylbutyrate. J Pediatr 2013;162:1228–34, 1234.e1.

17. Jalan R, Wright G, Davies NA, et al. L-Ornithine phenylacetate (OP): a novel treatment for hyperammonemia and hepatic encephalopathy. Med Hypotheses 2007; 69:1064–9.
18. Ventura-Cots M, Arranz JA, Simon-Talero M, et al. Safety of ornithine phenylacetate in cirrhotic decompensated patients: an open-label, dose-escalating, single-cohort study. J Clin Gastroenterol 2013;47:881–7.
19. Cordoba J, Ventura-Cots M. Drug-induced removal of nitrogen derivatives in urine: a new concept whose time has come. Hepatology 2014;59:764–6.
20. Shoji T, Wada A, Inoue K, et al. Prospective randomized study evaluating the efficacy of the spherical adsorptive carbon AST-120 in chronic kidney disease patients with moderate decrease in renal function. Nephron Clin Pract 2007;105:c99–107.
21. Schulman G, Agarwal R, Acharya M, et al. A multicenter, randomized, double-blind, placebo-controlled, dose-ranging study of AST-120 (Kremezin) in patients with moderate to severe CKD. Am J Kidney Dis 2006;47:565–77.
22. Sanaka T, Sugino N, Teraoka S, et al. Therapeutic effects of oral sorbent in undialyzed uremia. Am J Kidney Dis 1988;12:97–103.
23. Owada A, Nakao M, Koike J, et al. Effects of oral adsorbent AST-120 on the progression of chronic renal failure: a randomized controlled study. Kidney Int Suppl 1997;63:S188–90.
24. Shen B, Pardi DS, Bennett AE, et al. The efficacy and tolerability of AST-120 (spherical carbon adsorbent) in active pouchitis. Am J Gastroenterol 2009;104:1468–74.
25. Hiraishi M. The effect of oral adsorbent on surgically induced hepatic failure. Jpn J Surg 1987;17:517–27.
26. Pockros P, Hassanein T, Vierling J, et al. Phase 2, multicenter, randomized study of AST-120 (spherical carbon adsorbent) vs. lactulose in the treatment of low-grade hepatic encephalopathy (HE). J Hepatol 2009;50:S43–4 [Parallel Session 12: Cirrhosis and liver failure].
27. Bosoi CR, Parent-Robitaille C, Anderson K, et al. AST-120 (spherical carbon adsorbent) lowers ammonia levels and attenuates brain edema in bile duct-ligated rats. Hepatology 2011;53:1995–2002.
28. Kundra A, Jain A, Banga A, et al. Evaluation of plasma ammonia levels in patients with acute liver failure and chronic liver disease and its correlation with the severity of hepatic encephalopathy and clinical features of raised intracranial tension. Clin Biochem 2005;38:696–9.
29. Bajaj JS, Sheikh MY, Chojkier M, et al. AST-120 (spherical carbon adsorbent) in covert hepatic encephalopathy: results of the astute trial. J Hepatol 2013;58: S63–227 [abstract: 190].
30. Hassanein TI, Tofteng F, Brown RS Jr, et al. Randomized controlled study of extracorporeal albumin dialysis for hepatic encephalopathy in advanced cirrhosis. Hepatology 2007;46:1853–62.
31. Hill K, Hu KQ, Cottrell A, et al. Charcoal-based hemodiabsorption liver support for episodic type C hepatic encephalopathy. Am J Gastroenterol 2003;98:2763–70.
32. Rahimi RS, Singal AG, Cuthbert JA, et al. Lactulose vs polyethylene glycol 3350-electrolyte solution for treatment of overt hepatic encephalopathy: the HELP randomized clinical trial. JAMA Intern Med 2014;174:1727–33.
33. Hammer HF, Santa Ana CA, Schiller LR, et al. studies of osmotic diarrhea induced in normal subjects by ingestion of polyethylene glycol and lactulose. J Clin Invest 1989;84:1056–62.

Treatment of Overt Hepatic Encephalopathy

Norman L. Sussman, MD

KEYWORDS

- Hepatic encephalopathy • Cirrhosis • Portal hypertension • Portosystemic shunt
- Ammonia

KEY POINTS

- Hepatic encephalopathy (HE) is caused by a combination of liver failure and portosystemic shunting.
- Any episode of HE may signal an important precipitating event; always consider infection, gastrointestinal bleeding, constipation, and metabolic derangements.
- HE is associated with an elevated blood ammonia concentration.
  - ○ Factors other than ammonia may contribute to HE, but remain to be defined.
  - ○ The actual blood ammonia concentration correlates poorly with clinical findings – serial monitoring is rarely useful.
  - ○ All current medical therapies are thought to work by reducing blood ammonia.
  - ○ Current drugs approved for managing HE are non-absorbable disaccharides and non-absorbable antibiotics.
- HE is associated with excess mortality beyond the Model for End-Stage Liver Disease score.
- Patients with HE should be considered for orthotopic liver transplantation.
- Investigational agents increase flux through the urea cycle or increase urinary excretion of other ammonia-containing compounds.

INTRODUCTION

Hepatic encephalopathy (HE) is a reversible impairment of neuropsychiatric function, usually caused by a combination of portosystemic shunting and impaired hepatic function. Cases of HE caused by a large shunt in the absence of cirrhosis are known as type B, and are considerably less common. The consequences and cost of HE are substantial; a recent study of patients in the United States reported 22,931 hospitalizations in 2009 with an average length of stay of 8.5 days at a cost of $63,108 per case and a mortality rate of about 15%.[1] A 10-year study of patients who were listed for orthotopic liver transplantation reported a significantly higher mortality among patients

The author has nothing to disclose.
Baylor College of Medicine and Baylor-St. Luke's Medical Center, Division of Abdominal Transplantation, 6620 Main Street #1425, Houston, TX 77030, USA
E-mail address: normans@bcm.edu

Clin Liver Dis 19 (2015) 551–563
http://dx.doi.org/10.1016/j.cld.2015.04.005
1089-3261/15/$ – see front matter © 2015 Elsevier Inc. All rights reserved.

liver.theclinics.com

with HE; the 90-day wait-list mortality was significantly higher among patients with advanced HE compared with those with low-grade or no HE (24.4% vs 6.8% vs 3.5%, respectively; *P*<.001). When stratified by Model for End-Stage Liver Disease (MELD) score, patients with severe HE had a 90-day wait-list mortality similar to that of nonencephalopathic patients with MELD scores 6 to 7 points higher (**Fig. 1**).[2]

The individual contributions of liver dysfunction and portosystemic shunting are not easily separated, and the basis of HE is incompletely understood. HE is frequently ascribed to excess activity of γ-aminobutyric acid-ergic (inhibitory) neurons in the brain in response to nitrogenous overload. The basis of treatment has therefore centered on reducing blood ammonia concentrations. This empiric approach works fairly well, but the role of blood ammonia concentration as a single agent is frequently overemphasized in clinical practice. Although beyond the scope of this review, other factors such as cerebral blood flow and oxygen extraction may be affected in patients with HE, and do not seem to be related to blood ammonia or the cerebral metabolic rate of blood ammonia.[3]

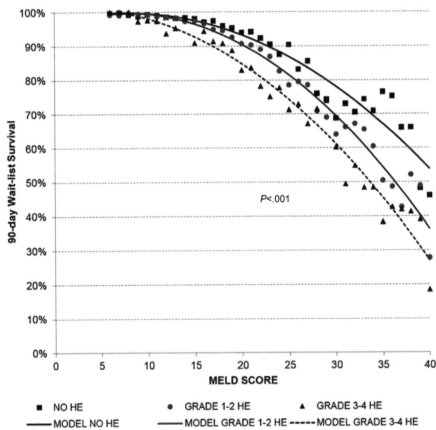

Fig. 1. Ninety-day wait-list survival stratified by Model for End-Stage Liver Disease (MELD) score and severity of hepatic encephalopathy (HE). The presence of advanced (grade 3–4) HE increases mortality by the equivalent of 6 to 7 points when compared with patients without HE. (*From* Wong RJ, Gish RG, Ahmed A. Hepatic encephalopathy is associated with significantly increased mortality among patients awaiting liver transplantation. Liver Transpl 2014;20:1459; with permission.)

Current thinking about HE includes a subclinical syndrome (minimal HE) that is evident only on neuropsychiatric testing, and has led to the concept of HE as a continuum of brain function from normal to subtle impairment to markedly abnormal.[4,5] HE is also divided into type A (associated with acute liver failure), type B (HE related to portosystemic shunting in the absence of parenchymal liver disease), and type C (HE in the presence of cirrhosis and portal hypertension).[6] Comments in this article are confined to overt HE related to chronic liver disease. For the purposes of this article, HE refers to overt (clinically apparent) HE unless otherwise specified.

CLINICAL FEATURES

The clinical features of overt HE include sleep–wake disturbances, personality changes, altered mentation, and a flapping tremor (asterixis). The appearance of any single finding, the severity of the individual components, and the appearance of additional features vary widely. The most frequently used tool in research and clinical practice is the West Haven scale, which focuses entirely on mental status.[7] The scale ranges from trivial lack of awareness or alteration in sleep–wake cycle (grade I) to coma (grade IV).[7]

MANAGEMENT OF HEPATIC ENCEPHALOPATHY

We consider the management of HE in 3 categories (**Table 1**).

- Ensure patient safety
  - The initial evaluation must include an assessment of patient safety. If the patient is a danger to self or others, hospitalization should be arranged.

Table 1
Stepwise approach to managing overt HE

Factor	Details
Ensure patient safety	• Admit to hospital if the patient is not safe at home • Assess whether patient can drive

Check for precipitating factors and alternative diagnoses	• Infections – spontaneous bacterial peritonitis, bacteremia, urinary tract infection, pulmonary infection, cellulitis, dental abscess
	• Drug use (prescription or nonprescription), especially alcohol, narcotics and benzodiazepines
	• Metabolic derangements
	  ○ Hypoglycemia or hyperglycemia
	  ○ Hyponatremia
	  ○ Hypokalemia with or without alkalosis
	  ○ Dehydration with or without acute kidney injury
	• Constipation
	• Gastrointestinal bleeding
	• Wernicke encephalopathy (chronic alcoholism)
	• Primary brain problem (injury, stroke, seizure)

Treat	• Treat infection as soon as suspected or recognized • Treat the precipitating factor if possible (eg, gastrointestinal bleeding, dehydration) • Correct blood sugar, electrolyte, and acid–base disturbances • Purgatives – lactulose or bowel preparation if constipated • Nonabsorbable antibiotics (rifaximin, neomycin) • Experimental therapies (branched chain amino acids, glycerol phenylbutyrate, ornithine phenylacetate)

- Patients who are admitted to the hospital may be at risk for various hazards including aspiration and falls; an appropriate level of observation is essential.
- Patients who are sent home with HE should have a caregiver who is able to prevent injury, monitor the patient's mental status, and ensure compliance with medication.
- Evaluate and treat precipitating factors, if present
  - A number of conditions and metabolic derangements may precipitate or contribute to HE; the most common are listed in **Table 1**. Bacterial infections are the most common identifiable precipitating factor, but the other problems occur with sufficient frequency to warrant investigation in the appropriate setting. Management of factors like spontaneous bacterial peritonitis, hypoglycemia, gastrointestinal bleeding, acute kidney injury, acid–base and electrolyte disorders, and inappropriate drug use are beyond the scope of this review, and will not be discussed further; however, they are largely addressed in several recent reviews.[8,9]
- Treat hepatic encephalopathy
  - Treatment options for HE are limited. Only 2 drugs are approved in the United States, namely, lactulose and rifaximin. Both drugs address ammonia production, and are discussed elsewhere in this article. Additional potential agents are also discussed.

INITIAL ASSESSMENT AND MANAGEMENT

The initial assessment of the patient with HE should include chronicity (how long have symptoms been recognized?), frequency (is this the first presentation, or has the patient had recurrent episodes?), and severity (using the West Haven scale). Patients with severe impairment or those who live in a poorly monitored environment should be admitted to a facility where they can be safely observed and treated. Ambulatory patients with mild HE may actually be more challenging. These patients frequently fail to recognize their impairment, and they may disagree with their families about the extent or even the existence of impaired mentation. Even worse, patients may arrive unaccompanied, having driven themselves to their appointment. The provider may have trouble determining the extent of impairment, and may face the practical and ethical dilemma of letting a potentially impaired driver back on the road.

Driving impairment in patients with even minimal HE is well-documented,[10] and self-assessment with driving simulation may help patients to understand their disability.[11] Furthermore, a 5-year study demonstrated the cost effectiveness of psychometric testing and targeted treatment with lactulose.[12] Patients with mild overt HE are similarly (or more seriously) impaired, and should be strongly discouraged from driving. The legal issue surrounding HE has been addressed several times—only 6 states require providers to report medically impaired drivers, and HE is not mentioned specifically in any state.[13,14] Furthermore, the most recent survey found no completed lawsuits against physicians or patients for motor vehicle accidents associated with driving impairment caused by HE.[13] Despite these facts, the authors concluded that the responsibility of identifying potentially hazardous drivers might still lie with the physician.

Precipitating Factors

The initial assessment of the patient with HE should include evaluation for alternative causes of encephalopathy and precipitating factors of HE. In patients with recurrent

HE, infections and metabolic derangements are quite common, and intracranial events are rare. Patients who are admitted through the emergency department frequently get a CT of the brain. A large, retrospective Danish study identified patients with intracranial hemorrhage, and found that cirrhosis, alcoholic cirrhosis, and noncirrhotic alcoholic liver disease were overrepresented in this group (5- to 7-fold increased risk of intracranial hemorrhage compared with other populations).[15] This may be a misleading interpretation of risk. A more useful analysis was a 10-year retrospective study of 426 patients with cirrhosis and head CT that showed that patients with a fall, trauma, focal neurologic signs, or a history of intracranial hemorrhage had an intracranial bleed in 13 of 146 cases (9%). On the other hand, patients who presented with altered mental status, headache, or fever had an intracranial event in 1 of 316 cases (<1%). The number needed to scan for each positive result depended on the indication: focal neurologic deficit = 9, fall or trauma = 20, altered mental status in the absence of these factors = 316.[16] We do not recommend routine head CT in the absence of clinical suspicion as defined in this recent article.

Nutrition and Branched Chain Amino Acids

Protein calorie malnutrition (PCM) is a common finding and an indicator of poor prognosis in patients with cirrhosis.[17] The basis of PCM is multifactorial, and includes poor protein intake (frequently recommended by a misinformed health care provider), episodes of inflammation and sepsis, gastrointestinal bleeding, and frequent paracentesis or thoracentesis.[18] A diet that fails to keep up with these losses rapidly leads to PCM and muscle wasting (sarcopenia). Both PCM and sarcopenia are overlooked frequently, especially in obese patients or those with fluid retention—in both cases body mass index fails to classify patients correctly.

Skeletal muscle is the second largest site of ammonia metabolism after the liver. In well-nourished cirrhotic patients, muscles synthesize glutamate from branched chain amino acids (BCAA; valine, leucine, and isoleucine). Glutamate is then condensed with ammonia to form glutamine (GLN) using GLN synthase as a catalyst.[19] This pathway explains a number of facts about cirrhotic patients, including the lower concentration of BCAA in serum, the potential for patients with muscle wasting to have worse HE, and the theoretic advantage of feeding with a diet enriched in BCAA. Protein should be divided between at least 4 meals every day, and patients should take a late evening snack to reduce protein breakdown during the overnight fast.[20–22] Vegetable protein may be used in patients who cannot tolerate animal protein. Protein restriction should never be recommended.

BCAAs in general, and leucine in particular, reduce protein degradation through direct stimulation of the mammalian target of rapamycin.[23] The addition of leucine to dietary supplements may promote protein synthesis and reduce blood ammonia levels. This in turn may enable patients to consume adequate dietary protein without worsening HE. BCAA may also compete with aromatic amino acids for blood–brain barrier transporters, and thus reduce the formation of false neurotransmitters. A systematic review of 8 trials (382 patients) and recalculated outcomes in 4 trials (255 patients) showed improved mental status in both minimal and overt HE, but no effect on survival or parameters of nutrition.[24]

A recent review raised a concern about the use of BCAA because GLN may be broken down in the intestine and kidney, thus releasing ammonia. This author recommended the concomitant administration of α-ketoglutarate to inhibit GLN breakdown in the intestine, and/or phenylbutyrate to enhance GLN excretion in the kidneys.[19] The role of phenylbutyrate is discussed elsewhere in this article.

MEDICAL THERAPY FOR OVERT HEPATIC ENCEPHALOPATHY

In addition to the steps discussed, HE should be treated with medication. Two drugs are approved in the United States, namely, lactulose and rifaximin.

Lactulose

Lactulose and lactitol are nonabsorbable disaccharides. Of the two, only lactulose is available in the United States. Although a Cochrane review found insufficient evidence to either support or refute the use of these agents,[25] they remain the most commonly prescribed medication for acute and recurrent HE, and are recommended in the practice guidelines put out jointly by American Association for the Study of Liver Diseases (AASLD) and European Association for the Study of the Liver (EASL).[7] An observational trial of 231 patients admitted to hospital with grade 2 to 3 HE reported that 78% responded to lactulose within 10 days of admission—the factors associated with nonresponse were lower blood pressure, higher MELD score, and a concomitant diagnosis of hepatocellular carcinoma.[26] Patients who are admitted for severe HE should have their lactulose dose reduced to maintenance levels once they have had several bowel movements. We use lactulose enemas in patients who are at risk for aspiration although objective evidence for this approach is lacking.

Preemptive lactulose use in patients who have never experienced HE is not recommended currently, although a study of asymptomatic cirrhotic patients demonstrated a marked reduction in symptomatic HE over the ensuing year (11% in patients on lactulose vs 28% in controls; $P = .02$).[27] Preemptive lactulose, with or without psychometric testing, was also cost effective in an analysis of patients with minimal HE.[12]

The mechanisms by which lactulose improves HE are thought to include its purgative action and alterations in colonic luminal pH with consequent changes in colonic bacteria and ammonia concentration.[28] The change in the gut microbiota is presumed, but difficult to prove.[29] The independent benefit of colonic cleansing alone was demonstrated in a randomized trial comparing polyethylene glycol 3350-electrolyte solution with lactulose in cirrhotic patients admitted to hospital for HE. This study showed similar improvements in HE in the 2 arms.[30]

Patients who present with an index episode of HE should be evaluated for ongoing maintenance therapy—so-called secondary prophylaxis. If the precipitating factor has resolved and the patient's status has improved materially (eg, variceal bleeding has been controlled, sepsis has been treated, or the patient has stopped consuming alcohol), observation may be appropriate.[7] In the absence of this type of improvement, secondary prophylaxis should be considered; we recommend lactulose 20 to 60 mL/d in divided doses to achieve 2 to 3 bowel movements daily. Patients and their caregivers should be counseled to prevent both underdosing and overdosing; chronic diarrhea may be detrimental because of the accompanying electrolyte and acid–base disturbances. A study by Bajaj and colleagues[31] showed that nearly one-half of HE recurrences after a first episode were related to either nonadherence or overdose. A randomized, unblinded trial of patients after an initial episode of HE reported a readmission rate of about 20% in patients who took lactulose versus about 47% in patients who did not.[32] The same group also reported the superiority of lactulose or probiotics over no treatment.[33] Readmission for other causes and death rate were similar in all groups. Not surprisingly, abnormal psychometric tests were common after recovery from HE, and the risk of recurrent HE was associated significantly with 2 or more abnormal psychometric tests after recovering from the initial episode of HE.

Rifaximin

Rifaximin is a nonabsorbable antibiotic that has very low systemic absorption and a high barrier to resistance. These characteristics make it superior to the historic alternatives used for HE, neomycin, metronidazole, and oral vancomycin.[34] A metaanalysis that compared nonabsorbable disaccharides with rifaximin found them to be equally effective, with no difference in the frequency of diarrhea, but improvement in abdominal pain in the rifaximin group.[35]

With 2 modestly effective agents available to treat HE, the natural question was whether a combination of the 2 agents might yield a superior outcome. A pivotal study by Bass and colleagues[36] on the prevention of recurrent HE showed that rifaximin, usually in combination with lactulose, was superior in maintaining freedom from HE (22% vs 46%) and reduced the risk of being hospitalized (14% vs 46%) over the 6 months of the study. Similarly, Sharma and colleagues[37] reported on 120 patients who were hospitalized with severe liver disease (mean MELD score, 24.6 ± 4.2) and overt HE (grade 2, 18%; grade 3, 33%; grade 4, 48%). Patients were randomized to dual therapy (lactulose plus rifaximin) or lactulose monotherapy. Two benefits were seen in the dual therapy arm; fewer deaths (7 vs 17) and shorter hospital stays (5.8 ± 3.4 vs 8.2 ± 4.6 days; $P = .001$).

An open-label extension of the Bass study[36] examined the safety of continuous rifaximin for 24 months. After a median duration of 427 days and 511 person-years of exposure, the profile and rate of adverse events with long-term rifaximin were similar to those in the original randomized control trial.[38] They also saw no increase in the rate of infections, including with *Clostridium difficile*, or development of bacterial antibiotic resistance. Another interesting analysis of the extension study examined patients who received placebo in the randomized trial, and were subsequently switched to rifaximin. More than 65% of the patients who experienced an episode of HE during the initial trial were protected from recurrent HE in the open-label extension. The number needed to treat to prevent an episode of HE was 3, very similar to the 4 needed in the initial trial.[39]

Treatment guidelines do not comment on use of a single agent versus 2 agents. We generally start lactulose as monotherapy in patients with mild HE, and add rifaximin if they have breakthrough HE. Rifaximin monotherapy is unproven, but may be used in patients who are unable to take lactulose (eg, patients with chronic diarrhea).

New and Experimental Agents

Probiotics

The effectiveness of lactulose and rifaximin suggest that altering gut flora to a non–urease-producing population may be effective in managing HE. Probiotics are not an accepted therapy for HE, but a study of primary prophylaxis showed that overt encephalopathy occurred in more controls than treated patients ($P<.05$; hazard ratio for controls vs probiotic group, 2.1; 95% CI, 1.31–6.53). As in previous studies from this group, abnormal psychometric testing correlated with the development of HE.[40] A different study randomized 130 patients who had recovered from an episode of HE to receive either a proprietary probiotic formulation (VSL#3, CD Pharma, New Delhi, India) or placebo. The probiotic group had a lower incidence of breakthrough HE although this did not reach statistical significance (35% in the probiotic group vs 52% in the placebo group; hazard ratio, 0.65; 95% CI, 0.38–1.11; $P = .12$).[41] We do not feel that the available data support the use of probiotics.

Zinc

Low zinc has been reported in cases of HE, leading to the theory that zinc supplementation might prove therapeutic. A metaanalysis of 4 trials (n = 233) found documented improvement in the number connection test in 3 trials, but episodes of HE were not reduced in 2 trials (n = 169).[42] Zinc replacement is not harmful, but it does not seem to have a place in the management of HE.

Alternative Methods of Ammonia Excretion

A number of compounds increase ammonia clearance by diverting it through alternative excretion pathways. These compounds (ammonia scavengers) were developed initially to treat urea cycle defects, enzyme deficiencies in which ammonia clearance is severely limited by the inability to form urea. The compounds include sodium benzoate, sodium phenylbutyrate (SPB), glycerol phenylbutyrate (GPB), L-ornithine L-aspartate (LOLA), and ornithine phenylacetate (OPA).

Sodium benzoate

Sodium benzoate increases ammonia clearance through glycine conjugation, and is combined with sodium phenylacetate (Ammonul, Ucyclyd Pharma, Scottsdale, AZ, USA) or SPB (Buphenyl, Ucyclyd Pharma) for treating urea cycle defects.[43] The need for intravenous administration and the high sodium content suggest that sodium benzoate will not be useful in treating HE.

Sodium phenylbutyrate and glycerol phenylbutyrate

SPB is converted to phenylbutyric acid and then to phenylacetate, which combines with GLN to form phenylacetylglutamine, which is excreted in the urine (**Fig. 2**). The sodium load of SPB makes it less desirable in patients with cirrhosis. GPB is an alternative to SPB; it is a liquid triglyceride precursor of phenylbutyric acid that is taken orally and has proven safe in normal and cirrhotic subjects.[44] A phase II clinical trial showed that GBP lowered serum ammonia levels and reduced the proportion of patients who experienced HE as well as time to first event and total HE events.[45] GPB is available as Ravicti (Hyperion Therapeutics, Inc, Brisbane, CA, USA). It is approved for restricted use in hyperammonemia, and is expected to proceed to phase III testing for HE.

Ornithine phenylacetate

As for GPB, phenylacetate levels can be increased by administering OPA. The effect is the same as for GPB; phenylacetate binds to GLN and is excreted in urine as phenylacetylglutamine, trapping 2 molecules of ammonia. A clinical trial in patients with gastrointestinal bleeding showed a 37% decrease in serum ammonia at day 3 with 32% of administered OPA recovered in the urine as phenylacetylglutamine.[46] Further trials are needed to determine whether OPA has a role in managing refractory HE.

L-Ornithine L-aspartate (LOLA)

Both ornithine and aspartate are substrates of the urea cycle, and seem to stimulate enzyme activity in residual hepatocytes, even in decompensated cirrhosis. LOLA has a dual action: increased production of urea by increasing carbamyl phosphate synthetase in periportal hepatocytes and increased production of GLN by increasing GLN synthetase in pericentral hepatocytes and skeletal muscle.[47] A metaanalysis of 8 randomized, controlled trials with 646 patients showed that LOLA was significantly more effective in controlling HE and minimal HE, and significantly reduced fasting ammonia levels.[48] LOLA was reported recently to have no effect on minimal HE, but to reduce episodes of overt HE.[49]

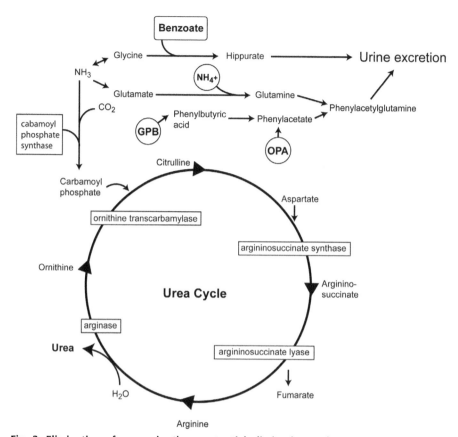

Fig. 2. Elimination of ammonia: three potential elimination pathways. Ammonia is normally eliminated as urea via the urea cycle. L-ornithine L-aspartate (LOLA) increases activity of the urea cycle. Patients who lack one of the enzymes of the urea cycle (shown in boxes) accumulate ammonia. These patients may be treated with ammonia scavengers that increase ammonia excretion in the urine. Benzoate promotes ammonia excretion as hippurate (one NH_4^+ per molecule). Phenylacetate (given as ornithine phenylacetate [OPA]) or its precursors, sodium phenylbutyrate (SPB) or glycerol phenylbutyrate (GPB) promote ammonia excretion as phenylacetylglutamine (two NH_4^+ per molecule).

EMBOLIZATION OF PORTOSYSTEMIC SHUNTS

The importance of portosystemic shunting in the generation of HE is demonstrated by the frequent appearance of HE after insertion of a transjugular intrahepatic portosystemic shunt (TIPS), and by the reversal of HE following occlusion of the same TIPS.[50] Similarly, patients with or without cirrhosis may have a dominant spontaneous portosystemic shunt (frequently splenorenal) that diverts venous blood from the portal system. These usually occur in the presence of cirrhosis, and may persist after placement of TIPS. We have seen patients with spontaneous splenorenal shunts in the absence of cirrhosis, but we find no similar reports in the literature. Limited experience suggests that these patients may benefit from occlusion of large shunts. A study of 7 patients treated with balloon-occluded retrograde transvenous obliteration demonstrated improved encephalopathy and serum ammonia in all 8

(1 patient required a second session of balloon-occluded retrograde transvenous obliteration).[51] A retrospective study of 17 patients with HE demonstrated a lower incidence of HE (40% vs 80%, $P = .02$) after coil embolization compared with controls.[52] Their claim of improved survival in a subset of patients is less believable, but deserves further study. Based on these results, many interventional radiologists embolize large portosystemic shunts at the time of TIPS placement.[52] Similarly, patients with HE out of proportion to other signs of portal hypertension (eg, the absence of ascites or varices), should undergo high-quality contrast imaging to examine for obvious anatomic portosystemic shunts.

ARTIFICIAL LIVER SUPPORT

Liver support devices are in development, but have not been tested adequately to recommend them in the treatment of HE.[53,54] A recent study of molecular adsorbents recirculating system (MARS; albumin dialysis) in patients with acute-on-chronic liver failure showed a trend toward improved HE, although this did not attain significance.[55]

LIVER TRANSPLANTATION

Liver transplantation resolves both hepatic dysfunction and portal hypertension, and usually results in complete resolution of HE. HE does not necessarily correlate with MELD score, so patients with HE may be disadvantaged in the era of MELD-based organ allocation despite a serious impact of HE on productivity, health, and survival.

SUMMARY

HE is a frustrating condition with limited treatment options and a high associated mortality from liver failure. It is a substantial drain on social and medical resources because of the frequent need for hospital readmission and the need for a supervised home environment. Treatment options include medical therapy, all of which aim at reducing blood ammonia levels. Combinations of 2 medications seem to be additive, but not synergistic, raising concern that easier or more efficient methods of reducing ammonia concentrations may have limited efficacy. Large portosystemic shunts may contribute to HE, and embolization of these shunts may improve HE. Severe HE usually indicates the need for orthotopic liver transplantation although the presence of HE does not, in itself, increase the likelihood of orthotopic liver transplantation in the era of MELD-based organ allocation.

REFERENCES

1. Stepanova M, Mishra A, Venkatesan C, et al. In-hospital mortality and economic burden associated with hepatic encephalopathy in the United States from 2005 to 2009. Clin Gastroenterol Hepatol 2012;10:1034–41.e1.
2. Wong RJ, Gish RG, Ahmed A. Hepatic encephalopathy is associated with significantly increased mortality among patients awaiting liver transplantation. Liver Transpl 2014;20:1454–61.
3. Dam G, Keiding S, Munk OL, et al. Hepatic encephalopathy is associated with decreased cerebral oxygen metabolism and blood flow, not increased ammonia uptake. Hepatology 2013;57:258–65.
4. Randolph C, Hilsabeck R, Kato A, et al. Neuropsychological assessment of hepatic encephalopathy: ISHEN practice guidelines. Liver Int 2009;29:629–35.

5. Bajaj JS, Wade JB, Sanyal AJ. Spectrum of neurocognitive impairment in cirrhosis: implications for the assessment of hepatic encephalopathy. Hepatology 2009;50:2014–21.
6. Savlan I, Liakina V, Valantinas J. Concise review of current concepts on nomenclature and pathophysiology of hepatic encephalopathy. Medicina 2014;50: 75–81.
7. Vilstrup H, Amodio P, Bajaj J, et al. Hepatic encephalopathy in chronic liver disease: 2014 Practice Guideline by the American Association for the Study of Liver Diseases and the European Association for the Study of the Liver. Hepatology 2014;60:715–35.
8. Nusrat S, Khan MS, Fazili J, et al. Cirrhosis and its complications: evidence based treatment. World J Gastroenterol 2014;20:5442–60.
9. Peck-Radosavljevic M, Angeli P, Cordoba J, et al. Managing complications in cirrhotic patients. United European Gastroenterol J 2015;3:80–94.
10. Wein C, Koch H, Popp B, et al. Minimal hepatic encephalopathy impairs fitness to drive. Hepatology 2004;39:739–45.
11. Bajaj JS, Thacker LR, Heuman DM, et al. Driving simulation can improve insight into impaired driving skills in cirrhosis. Dig Dis Sci 2012;57:554–60.
12. Bajaj JS, Pinkerton SD, Sanyal AJ, et al. Diagnosis and treatment of minimal hepatic encephalopathy to prevent motor vehicle accidents: a cost-effectiveness analysis. Hepatology 2012;55:1164–71.
13. Cohen SM, Kim A, Metropulos M, et al. Legal ramifications for physicians of patients who drive with hepatic encephalopathy. Clin Gastroenterol Hepatol 2011;9:156–60 [quiz: e17].
14. Aschkenasy MT, Drescher MJ, Ratzan RM. Physician reporting of medically impaired drivers. J Emerg Med 2006;30:29–39.
15. Gronbaek H, Johnsen SP, Jepsen P, et al. Liver cirrhosis, other liver diseases, and risk of hospitalisation for intracerebral haemorrhage: a Danish population-based case-control study. BMC Gastroenterol 2008;8:16.
16. Donovan LM, Kress WL, Strnad LC, et al. Low likelihood of intracranial hemorrhage in patients with cirrhosis and altered mental status. Clin Gastroenterol Hepatol 2015;13:165–9.
17. Chadalavada R, Sappati Biyyani RS, Maxwell J, et al. Nutrition in hepatic encephalopathy. Nutr Clin Pract 2010;25:257–64.
18. Bemeur C, Desjardins P, Butterworth RF. Role of nutrition in the management of hepatic encephalopathy in end-stage liver failure. J Nutr Metab 2010;2010: 489823.
19. Holecek M. Branched-chain amino acids and ammonia metabolism in liver disease: therapeutic implications. Nutrition 2013;29:1186–91.
20. Swart GR, Zillikens MC, van Vuure JK, et al. Effect of a late evening meal on nitrogen balance in patients with cirrhosis of the liver. BMJ 1989;299:1202–3.
21. Holecek M. Ammonia and amino acid profiles in liver cirrhosis: effects of variables leading to hepatic encephalopathy. Nutrition 2015;31:14–20.
22. Tsien CD, McCullough AJ, Dasarathy S. Late evening snack: exploiting a period of anabolic opportunity in cirrhosis. J Gastroenterol Hepatol 2012;27:430–41.
23. Nishitani S, Ijichi C, Takehana K, et al. Pharmacological activities of branched-chain amino acids: specificity of tissue and signal transduction. Biochem Biophys Res Commun 2004;313:387–9.
24. Gluud LL, Dam G, Borre M, et al. Oral branched-chain amino acids have a beneficial effect on manifestations of hepatic encephalopathy in a systematic review with meta-analyses of randomized controlled trials. J Nutr 2013;143:1263–8.

25. Als-Nielsen B, Gluud LL, Gluud C. Nonabsorbable disaccharides for hepatic en-cephalopathy. Cochrane Database Syst Rev 2004;(2):CD003044.
26. Sharma P, Sharma BC, Sarin SK. Predictors of nonresponse to lactulose in pa-tients with cirrhosis and hepatic encephalopathy. Eur J Gastroenterol Hepatol 2010;22:526–31.
27. Sharma P, Sharma BC, Agrawal A, et al. Primary prophylaxis of overt hepatic encephalopathy in patients with cirrhosis: an open labeled randomized controlled trial of lactulose versus no lactulose. J Gastroenterol Hepatol 2012; 27:1329–35.
28. Romero-Gomez M, Montagnese S, Jalan R. Hepatic encephalopathy in patients with acute decompensation of cirrhosis and acute on chronic liver failure. J Hepatol 2015;62(2):437–47.
29. Bajaj JS. The role of microbiota in hepatic encephalopathy. Gut Microbes 2014;5: 397–403.
30. Rahimi RS, Singal AG, Cuthbert JA, et al. Lactulose vs polyethylene glycol 3350-electrolyte solution for treatment of overt hepatic encephalopathy: the help ran-domized clinical trial. JAMA Intern Med 2014;174:1727–33.
31. Bajaj JS, Sanyal AJ, Bell D, et al. Predictors of the recurrence of hepatic en-cephalopathy in lactulose-treated patients. Aliment Pharmacol Ther 2010;31: 1012–7.
32. Sharma BC, Sharma P, Agrawal A, et al. Secondary prophylaxis of hepatic en-cephalopathy: an open-label randomized controlled trial of lactulose versus placebo. Gastroenterology 2009;137:885–91, 891.e1.
33. Agrawal A, Sharma BC, Sharma P, et al. Secondary prophylaxis of hepatic en-cephalopathy in cirrhosis: an open-label, randomized controlled trial of lactulose, probiotics, and no therapy. Am J Gastroenterol 2012;107:1043–50.
34. Patidar KR, Bajaj JS. Antibiotics for the treatment of hepatic encephalopathy. Metab Brain Dis 2013;28:307–12.
35. Jiang Q, Jiang XH, Zheng MH, et al. Rifaximin versus nonabsorbable disaccha-rides in the management of hepatic encephalopathy: a meta-analysis. Eur J Gas-troenterol Hepatol 2008;20:1064–70.
36. Bass NM, Mullen KD, Sanyal A, et al. Rifaximin treatment in hepatic encephalop-athy. N Engl J Med 2010;362:1071–81.
37. Sharma BC, Sharma P, Lunia MK, et al. A randomized, double-blind, controlled trial comparing rifaximin plus lactulose with lactulose alone in treatment of overt hepatic encephalopathy. Am J Gastroenterol 2013;108:1458–63.
38. Mullen KD, Sanyal AJ, Bass NM, et al. Rifaximin is safe and well tolerated for long-term maintenance of remission from overt hepatic encephalopathy. Clin Gastroenterol Hepatol 2014;12:1390–7.e2.
39. Bajaj JS, Barrett AC, Bortey E, et al. Prolonged remission from hepatic encepha-lopathy with rifaximin: results of a placebo crossover analysis. Aliment Pharmacol Ther 2014;41(1):39–45.
40. Lunia MK, Sharma BC, Sharma P, et al. Probiotics prevent hepatic encephalop-athy in patients with cirrhosis: a randomized controlled trial. Clin Gastroenterol Hepatol 2014;12:1003–8.e1.
41. Dhiman RK, Rana B, Agrawal S, et al. Probiotic VSL#3 reduces liver disease severity and hospitalization in patients with cirrhosis: a randomized, controlled trial. Gastroenterology 2014;147:1327–37.e3.
42. Chavez-Tapia NC, Cesar-Arce A, Barrientos-Gutierrez T, et al. A systematic re-view and meta-analysis of the use of oral zinc in the treatment of hepatic enceph-alopathy. Nutr J 2013;12:74.

43. Misel ML, Gish RG, Patton H, et al. Sodium benzoate for treatment of hepatic encephalopathy. Gastroenterol Hepatol (N Y) 2013;9:219–27.
44. McGuire BM, Zupanets IA, Lowe ME, et al. Pharmacology and safety of glycerol phenylbutyrate in healthy adults and adults with cirrhosis. Hepatology 2010;51: 2077–85.
45. Rockey DC, Vierling JM, Mantry P, et al. Randomized, double-blind, controlled study of glycerol phenylbutyrate in hepatic encephalopathy. Hepatology 2014; 59:1073–83.
46. Ventura-Cots M, Arranz JA, Simon-Talero M, et al. Safety of ornithine phenylacetate in cirrhotic decompensated patients: an open-label, dose-escalating, single-cohort study. J Clin Gastroenterol 2013;47:881–7.
47. Jover-Cobos M, Khetan V, Jalan R. Treatment of hyperammonemia in liver failure. Curr Opin Clin Nutr Metab Care 2014;17:105–10.
48. Bai M, Yang Z, Qi X, et al. l-Ornithine-l-aspartate for hepatic encephalopathy in patients with cirrhosis: a meta-analysis of randomized controlled trials. J Gastroenterol Hepatol 2013;28:783–92.
49. Alvares-da-Silva MR, de Araujo A, Vicenzi JR, et al. Oral l-ornithine-l-aspartate in minimal hepatic encephalopathy: a randomized, double-blind, placebo-controlled trial. Hepatol Res 2014;44:956–63.
50. Kerlan RK Jr, LaBerge JM, Baker EL, et al. Successful reversal of hepatic encephalopathy with intentional occlusion of transjugular intrahepatic portosystemic shunts. J Vasc Interv Radiol 1995;6:917–21.
51. Mukund A, Rajesh S, Arora A, et al. Efficacy of balloon-occluded retrograde transvenous obliteration of large spontaneous lienorenal shunt in patients with severe recurrent hepatic encephalopathy with foam sclerotherapy: initial experience. J Vasc Interv Radiol 2012;23:1200–6.
52. An J, Kim KW, Han S, et al. Improvement in survival associated with embolisation of spontaneous portosystemic shunt in patients with recurrent hepatic encephalopathy. Aliment Pharmacol Ther 2014;39:1418–26.
53. Hassanein TI, Schade RR, Hepburn IS. Acute-on-chronic liver failure: extracorporeal liver assist devices. Curr Opin Crit Care 2011;17:195–203.
54. Sussman NL, Kelly JH. Artificial liver. Clin Gastroenterol Hepatol 2014;12:1439–42.
55. Banares R, Nevens F, Larsen FS, et al. Extracorporeal albumin dialysis with the molecular adsorbent recirculating system in acute-on-chronic liver failure: the RELIEF trial. Hepatology 2013;57:1153–62.

Diagnosis and Management of Hepatic Encephalopathy in Fulminant Hepatic Failure

Sudha Kodali, MD*, Brendan M. McGuire, MD

KEYWORDS

- Hepatic encephalopathy • Fulminant hepatic failure • Ammonia • Hyperammonemia

KEY POINTS

- Hepatic encephalopathy (HE) development in fulminant hepatic failure (FHF) is associated with a decrease in survival rates.
- Cerebral edema (CE) and intracranial pressure (ICP) are associated with elevated ammonia levels and are responsible for death in patients with FHF.
- Infection and the resulting inflammation can cause further worsening of HE in FHF patients.
- Ruling out other causes of altered mental status, identifying and correcting the trigger, and treatment should all be started simultaneously.
- The utility of lactulose and rifaximin for treating encephalopathy in FHF is unclear.

INTRODUCTION

HE is a neuropsychiatric syndrome due to hepatic dysfunction and portosystemic shunting.[1] In FHF, HE is primarily driven by hepatic dysfunction. In chronic liver disease, HE is primarily driven by portosystemic shunting. In FHF, CE leading to increased cerebral blood flow and intracranial hypertension (ICH) is one of the major causes of morbidity and mortality but in chronic liver disease ICH is rarely seen.[2,3] HE development in FHF signals a critical phase of illness.[4] HE is one of the most debilitating manifestations of FHF and, unless the underlying liver disease is successfully treated, is associated with poor survival.[5] The mortality rates in acute liver failure

The authors have nothing to disclose.
Department of Gastroenterology and Hepatology, University of Alabama at Birmingham, 1808 Seventh Avenue South, Birmingham, AL 35294-0012, USA
* Corresponding author.
E-mail address: skodali@uabmc.edu

(ALF) can be as high as 40% to 80% without a liver transplant.[2,6,7] CE and ICH secondary to elevated ammonia levels are responsible for death in up to 35% patients with FHF.[2] Such high mortality rates are not seen in patients with chronic liver failure.[8]

FHF has been classified based on symptom duration and by etiologies. The timing of HE in relation to jaundice has been classified as hyperacute (<7 days), acute (7–28 days), and subacute (4–26 weeks) FHF.[2,4,9] In addition, FHF has been classified by etiology, including viral infections, autoimmune disease, toxins (including drugs), metabolic causes, and ischemia. Sometimes a specific cause for FHF is not identified and these cases are classified as indeterminant.[2] Irrespective of the speed of FHF or the cause, all cases of FHF can progress in the severity of HE. The precipitating factor that usually drives HE in patients with FHF is elevated ammonia level plus another triggering factor resulting in neurochemical changes in the brain. Astrocytes in the brain are involved in detoxification of ammonia. Common additional triggering factors contributing to HE include infection, hyponatremia, hypoxemia, hypokalemia, and/or hypovolemia. In acetaminophen-induced ALF, there is a temporal association between acquisition of infection and subsequent progression of HE whereas in subjects with nonacetaminophen-induced ALF, the role of infection is less clear.[10] Infection and a systemic inflammatory response can cause worsening of HE in FHF.[4]

DEFINITION

HE is a neuropsychiatric syndrome due to hepatic dysfunction and caused by 2 mechanisms, hepatic dysfunction and portosystemic shunting.[9] Patients can present with symptoms ranging from mild psychometric testing abnormalities to alteration in behavior and coma.

SYMPTOM CRITERIA

- HE is classified broadly into minimal and overt HE.
- Patients with minimal HE present with normal mental and neurologic status but have abnormal results on psychometric testing.
- Patients with overt HE present clinically with an abnormal neuropsychiatric state.[11]

CLINICAL FINDINGS
Physical Examination

Patients can present with personality changes, such as apathy, irritability, and disinhibition. As the liver failure worsens, disorientation to time and space, inappropriate behavior, and acute state of confusion with agitation or somnolence, stupor, and, finally, coma can occur. The West Haven criteria are frequently used to assess the severity of HE. New-onset systemic hypertension, progression of HE, alterations in pupillary reactivity, abnormalities in oculovestibular reflexes, and decerebrate posturing may indicate the development of ICH in FHF patients.[12]

Rating Scale

The West Haven criteria, proposed by Conn and colleagues in 1977, grade mental status of a patient by assessing behavior, intellectual function, neuromuscular function, and altered consciousness. Although widely used, interobserver variability has been an issue with this test.[11] The West Haven criteria relies solely on the clinician's judgment to determine the presence and severity of HE. Grade 0 indicates no or minimal HE, with no overt neuropsychiatric or neurologic symptoms and no asterixis. Grade 1 is the trivial lack of awareness, shortened attention span, sleep disturbance, altered mood, slowed ability to perform mental tasks, and asterixis exhibited on physical examination. Grade 2 is lethargy or apathy, disorientation to time, amnesia of recent events, impaired simple computations, inappropriate behavior, slurred speech, and asterixis. Grade 3 is somnolence, confusion, disorientation to place, bizarre behavior, clonus, nystagmus, and positive Babinski sign. Asterixis is usually absent in grade 3. Grade 4 implies an unconscious patient who is comatose (**Table 1**).[11,13]

DIAGNOSTIC MODALITIES

Exclusion of other causes of encephalopathy is essential in the diagnosis of HE. Infection, hypoxemia, hypovolemia, and electrolyte abnormalities should always be ruled out along with subdural/intracerebral hemorrhage. Medication-related side effects always should be ruled out, because poor hepatic function alters hepatic detoxification.[11,14]

Laboratory Values

Serum ammonia levels
Elevated serum ammonia levels correlate with the severity of HE but usually do not alter the management and do not have a significant predictive value if less than 100 μg/dL. In ALF, serum ammonia levels of greater than 200 μg/dL are suggestive of ICH and have a poor prognostic significance.[15] Ammonia levels may not reflect the true severity of HE if the blood sample is not collected and transported appropriately. The blood sample should be drawn without using a tourniquet and transported within 20 minutes of the blood draw on ice.[11]

Psychometric Tests

Hepatic encephalopathy scoring algorithm
The HE scoring algorithm (HESA) combines clinical impressions with neuropsychological performances to characterize HE. This system is useful in assessing patients with low grades of HE, but its utility in FHF patients is unclear.

Psychometric hepatic encephalopathy score
The working party at the 1998 World Congress of Gastroenterology endorsed the psychometric HE score (PHES) as the gold standard for diagnosis of HE. It consists of 5 tests that can be conducted at the bedside, including number connection test A, number connection test B, symbol test, line tracing test, and serial dotting test. Attention, functioning, speed, and response inhibition impairments can be identified

Table 1	
West Haven classification of hepatic encephalopathy	
Grade 1	Despite oriented in time and space, the patient appears to have some cognitive/behavioral decay with respect to his or her standard on clinical examination or to the caregiver
Grade 2	Disoriented for time (at least 3 of the following are wrong: day of the month, day of the week, month, season, or year) ± the above mentioned symptoms
Grade 3	Disoriented also for space (at least 3 of the following wrongly reported: country, state [or region], city, or place) ± the above mentioned symptoms
Grade 4	Coma

by using these tests. The PHES is good for diagnosing subtle or minimal HE diagnosis, but it is not widely used in FHF because of lack of normative data and difficulty conducting the tests in grades 3 and 4 HE.

Repeatable battery for assessment of neurologic status
The repeatable battery for assessment of neurologic status (RBANS) is also a series of written tests and has been used in several clinical studies assessing cortical and subcortical components. Patients with HE perform worse on the subcortical domains. RBANS is good for diagnosing subtle or minimal HE diagnosis.

Computerized Neuropsychometric Tests

Inhibitory control test
The inhibitory control test is used for minimal HE and has high sensitivity. It is not widely used and is available only in a few centers.

Cognitive drug research system
The cognitive drug research (CRD) test has a good correlation with neuropsychometric tests. It is time consuming and not widely used.

ImPACT assessment system
The ImPACT test is a repeatable battery score that has been validated for assessment of neurologic status and measures fine motor skills in patients with concussions but has not been validated in patients with FHF.

Neurophysiologic Tests

Critical flicker frequency
The critical flicker frequency test is used in clinical trials, requires special equipment, and is not available in most centers.[1]

Electroencephalogram
Electroencephalogram (EEG) is commonly used for assessing brain activity in the evaluation of encephalopathy. It detects changes in cerebral activity. The results can be nonspecific and can be affected by metabolic factors.[1] The sensitivity of this test is variable, ranging from 40% to 100%, depending on different studies.[11]

Radiologic Imaging

Computed tomography scan of the head
Imaging of the head has traditionally been used to diagnose cerebrovascular accidents and is helpful to rule out other causes of altered mental status.[11] In addition, a noncontrasted CT scan of the head may show CE, compression of basal cisterns, hydrocephalus, mass effect, and midline shift, which indicate increased ICP, but the absence of these findings does not exclude CE.[12]

MRI of the head
MRI is used to diagnose CE in patients with HE.[11] Classic MRI abnormalities include high signal intensity in the globus pallidus on T1-weighted images, likely a reflection of increased tissue concentrations of manganese, and an elevated glutamine/glutamate peak coupled with decreased myo-inositol and choline signals on proton magnetic resonance spectroscopy, representing disturbances in cell volume homeostasis secondary to brain hyperammonemia.[16] Magnetization transfer ratio measurements, fast fluid-attenuated inversion-recovery sequences, and diffusion-weighted images can be used to detect white matter abnormalities, which reflect increased central nervous system ammonia concentration.[16]

Transcranial doppler

Transcranial Doppler (TCD) is a noninvasive technique that measures the velocity of blood flowing through the intracranial vessels and can provide information regarding cerebral blood flow and ICP.[12] Cerebral autoregulation is impaired in FHF and cerebral blood flow has been shown to correlate with ICP in FHF. In FHF, high cerebral blood flow has been associated with a poorer prognosis.[12] TCD can also be used serially to follow the response to treatment of ICH.

Optic nerve sheath diameter

The optic nerve has a sheath that is continuous with the dura mater of the brain. The subarachnoid space in the optic nerve sheath communicates with the cranial sub-arachnoid space and thus optic nerve sheath diameter (ONSD) can be influenced by changes in cerebrospinal fluid pressure in the cranial cavity. ONSD has been increasingly used for monitoring ICP in many clinical settings. ONSD is measured by an ultrasonic probe placed over the eyelid.[17,18] A linear correlation between ONSD and ICP measurement has been shown and a significant reduction of the ONSD occurred after drainage of cerebrospinal fluid. The suggested cutoff value of ONSD to predict ICP greater than 20 mm Hg was 5.2 mm (**Table 2**).[19]

PATHOLOGY

Understanding the pathophysiology of HE in FHF has been limited. High ammonia levels correlate in general with the degree of HE but more strongly with the presence of CE in FHF. Ammonia is also eliminated by kidneys and higher ammonia levels are seen with concomitant acute kidney injury.[20]

The development of brain swelling due to osmotic changes within the brain and loss of capillary integrity occurs more commonly in hyperacute settings and in young patients where adaptation to rapid changes in brain glutamine levels cannot take place. Thus, acetaminophen patients, typically under age 35, are at highest risk for brain edema. High levels of arterial ammonia have been shown to correlate well with development of CE, reinforcing the glutamine hypothesis.[21] Increases in ICP because of CE increase the risk of morbidity and mortality in patients with FHF.[3,21]

Ammonia (NH_3) is water soluble and, under normal conditions, exists as ammonium ion (NH_4^+). Glutamine from the gastrointestinal tract and kidneys is the source of ammonia that enters the portal circulation. Serum ammonia is normally converted to urea in the liver and excreted by the kidneys. Some ammonia is also used by skeletal

Table 2 Diagnostic tests	
Tests	**Serum Ammonia Level**
Psychometric tests	HESA PHES RBANS
Computerized psychometric tests	Inhibitory control test CDR system ImPACT assessment system
Neurophysiologic tests	Critical flicker frequency EEG
Radiologic imaging	CT scan of head MRI of head TCD ONSD

muscle for glutamine synthesis. In FHF, elevated ammonia levels occur because of the liver's inability to detoxify it. This can be exacerbated by coexisting renal failure. The high serum ammonia can cross the blood-brain barrier and trigger HE.

In the brain, ammonia is converted to glutamine in the astrocytes by glutamine synthetase. Glutamine is osmotically active and causes CE and an increase in ICP.[3] When the astrocytes are exposed to high levels of ammonia like in FHF, it causes sudden increased formation of glutamine. In recent years, a Trojan horse hypothesis has gained considerable attention.[3,22] According to this hypothesis, glutamine releases ammonia after entering the mitochondria and this process is catalyzed by phosphate-activated glutaminase.[3] In the mitochondria, ammonia induces oxidative and nitrosative stress by formation of free radicals. This leads to an apoptotic process called mitochondrial permeability transition (MPT), which is characterized by a sudden loss of inner membrane potential and cessation of mitochondrial ATP synthesis. High intracellular calcium ion levels and alterations in mitochondrial redox state and pH can contribute to MPT.[3,23] MPT can cause an increase in cell volume in astrocytes when exposed to high ammonia levels. In patients with FHF and HE, there is compromised oxidative metabolism most likely due to mitochondrial dysfunction and this correlates positively with glutamine concentrations. Glutamine, an excitatory neurotransmitter, causes confusion, agitation, seizures, and coma.[11,24]

There is an association between HE and infection. The components of systemic inflammatory response syndrome (SIRS) include heart rate greater than 90 beats per minute; fever greater than 100.4°F or less than 96.8°F; respiratory rate greater than 20 per minute or arterial $Paco_2$ less than 32 mm Hg; and leukocyte count greater than 12,000 μg/L or less than 4000 μg/L or greater than 10% immature (band) forms. Infected patients with progressive HE manifested more SIRS components than other infected patients.[25] A prospective study examined progression of HE in 227 patients with FHF and early HE on admission and noted a clear temporal association between infection and subsequent progression of HE in acetaminophen-induced FHF. The role of infection was less clear in nonacetaminophen-induced FHF. Although previous studies recommended routine antibiotic prophylaxis for all FHF patients, a recent large, observational study showed that antimicrobial prophylaxis did not reduce the incidence of bloodstream infection or mortality within 21 days of FHF.[26] Bloodstream infections were associated, however, with increased 21-day mortality in patients with FHF. Thus, routine use of antimicrobial prophylaxis in patients with FHF is not supported.[26]

Ischemic injury and impaired regulation of cerebral perfusion have also been implicated as causative factors for CE. Some risk factors for the development of CE in patients with FHF include high-grade HE (grade III or IV), high serum ammonia concentrations (>200 μmol/L), and requirement for vasopressor support or renal replacement therapy.[21]

DIAGNOSTIC DILEMMAS

Ruling out other causes of encephalopathy and identifying potential triggers that can worsen mental status in a patient with FHF should be a clinical priority.

- Rule out other causes of encephalopathy (**Box 1**).
- Identify potential triggers that can worsen mental status (**Box 2**).

MANAGEMENT

N-acetylcysteine is beneficial in nonacetaminophen FHF patients showing early (grades I/II) HE and increases survival among these patients without the need for liver

---

Box 1
Differential diagnosis of encephalopathy

Diabetic complications—hypoglycemia, ketoacidosis, hyperosmolar, lactic acidosis

Alcohol related—intoxication, withdrawal, Wernicke encephalopathy

Drugs—benzodiazepines, neuroleptics, opioids

Central nervous system infections

Electrolyte disturbances—hyponatremia, hypernatremia, hypercalcemia

Nonconvulsive epilepsy and postictal confusion

Psychiatric disorders

Intracranial bleeds and stroke

Organ failure

Dementia (primary and secondary)

Brain lesions—traumatic, neoplasms, normal pressure hydrocephalus

---

transplantation.[27] Thus, administration of *N*-acetylcysteine should be initiated early when a diagnosis of FHF is established. Management consisting of intensive care support should be initiated to address the various organ dysfunctions associated with FHF.[2] In addition, correction of the underlying factors that precipitate or aggravate the encephalopathy is recommended.

Management of Hepatic Encephalopathy

Lactulose
An osmotic laxative has been used for its ability to alter the colonic intraluminal pH and to decrease the uptake of glutamine and ammonia in the gastrointestinal lumen.[28–30] There is a lack of data regarding its use in FHF patients.[31] Abdominal distention can also obscure the operative field and precipitate megacolon, hence complicating liver transplant surgery.[31,32]

Box 2
Identify precipitating factors

Gastrointestinal bleeding

Infections

Superimposed hepatocyte injury

Prior portal decompression procedure

Diuretic overdose

Electrolyte disturbance

Constipation

Infections

Dehydration

Anesthesia

Neomycin

The antibiotic neomycin inhibits mucosal glutaminase in the gastrointestinal lumen and reduces ammonia production in the gut lumen.[33] It acts by inhibiting the growth of bacteria that produce urease. Because of renal toxicity and ototoxicity, it is rarely used in FHF.[11,34]

Rifaximin

Rifaximin, a poorly absorbed antibiotic, is increasingly used for empiric therapy of HE in patients with chronic liver disease. In a randomized, double-blind, placebo-controlled trial, prolonged remission rates and significantly reduced risk of hospitalization were evident in patients with chronic liver disease and HE treated with rifaximin.[35] It is well tolerated by patients, with minimal side effects and drug interactions.[11,30,35] There are insufficient data to support its use in FHF.[34]

Nutrition

FHF patients are in a hypercatabolic state, and in addition to airway support and medical management of various organ dysfunctions, addressing their nutritional requirements is crucial. In these patients, nasogastric tube feeding using a polymeric standard formula should be the first-line approach; parenteral nutrition (PN) giving glucose, fat, amino acids, vitamins, and trace elements is initiated when enteral nutrition is insufficient or impracticable.[36] In 2009, the European Society for Clinical Nutrition and Metabolism recommended that PN is safe and improves mental state in patients with cirrhosis and severe HE. Perioperative (including liver transplantation) PN is safe and reduces the rate of complications. In FHF, PN is a safe second-line option to adequately feed patients in whom enteral nutrition is insufficient or impossible.[37] Branched-chain amino acids and vegetable-based protein diets have been studied for management of HE in patients with cirrhosis. Their use has shown to improve the recovery time of HE in addition to reducing hospitalization rates and length of hospital stay.[11,38] There are no clear recommendations or consensus regarding their use or benefit in FHF.[39]

Management of Cerebral Edema

The first step is to treat factors that can worsen CE like hyponatremia, fluid overload, hypoxia, fever, seizures, endotracheal suction, frequent movement of patient, any kind of stimulation, and hypercapnea.[2] Elevation of the head of the bed to 30°, maintenance of a neutral neck position, endotracheal intubation, minimizing painful stimuli, and control of arterial hypertension reduce the risk of increasing CE.[40] Propofol is commonly used for sedation given its rapid onset of action and because it may protect from intracerebral hemorrhage. Adequate pain control is crucial and fentanyl is the preferred agent of choice.[2]

ICP monitoring should be considered in patients who are evaluated for liver transplant and have deep coma grade (ie grade 4 HE). The response to various interventions for reducing ICP can be assessed with ICP monitoring. The goal of therapy in FHF is to maintain ICP less than 20 mm Hg and cerebral perfusion pressure (CPP) greater than 60 mm Hg. Sustained increased ICP preoperative, ICP greater than 20 mm Hg, and CPP less than 40 mm Hg for greater than 2 hours have correlated with severe neurologic complications after liver transplantation.[2] Many liver transplant programs use ICP monitoring to exclude patients for liver transplant. ONSD is an alternative to ICP monitoring. It is a surrogate marker for ICP and monitoring is a safe and noninvasive modality for checking for acute elevations in ICP in patients with FHF with HE.[41]

Management of Elevated Intracranial Pressure

- Hypertonic saline reduces ICH by osmotic and nonosmotic mechanisms.[42] It is recommended to administer hypertonic saline intravenously while carefully monitoring the serum sodium levels. Hypernatremic seizures are the feared complications of this treatment.[2]
- Mannitol is an osmotic agent that reduces ICP by drawing water from the brain parenchyma into the intravascular space. It works well if the ICP is less than 60 mm Hg at a dose of 0.5 to 1 g/kg intravenously.[43] If serum osmolality test is greater than 320 mOsm/L, mannitol is of minimal benefit. In patients with renal failure, mannitol loses its efficacy, and to be able to use it for reducing ICP, hemofiltration can be used, which also helps reduce ICP.[44]
- Hypothermia by cooling to a core temperature of 32°C to 35°C reduces ICP by lowering arterial ammonia levels and brain energy metabolism. Low core temperature also reverses systemic inflammatory reactions and improves cardiovascular hemodynamics by increasing mean arterial pressure.[2,45] Observational studies and a meta-analysis using hypothermia in patients without liver disease have strongly suggested an increased risk of pneumonia and sepsis in hypothermic patients compared with controls.[46] A retrospective cohort analysis of patients with ALF did not, however, show any difference in rates of tracheal and blood stream infections in hypothermic patients compared with controls.[26]
- Hyperventilation (Paco$_2$ 30–35 mm Hg) reduces ICP and can be used short term but, if used over prolonged periods of time, can cause vasoconstriction and worsen cerebral hypoxia secondary to hypoperfusion.[2,47]
- Barbiturates reduce brain oxygen utilization and are effective in lowering ICP but can cause arterial hypotension and negative inotropic effects and hence are used sparingly.[2,45]
- In patients with FHF, hepatectomy and temporary portocaval shunting can be used as a bridge to transplant in patients with elevated ICP. The necrotic liver is the source of inflammatory mediators, which can augment cerebral perfusion and potentially worsen the ICP.[2]

POTENTIAL FUTURE THERAPIES

Several liver support devices have been used for FHF patients with limited to no success. This is because the liver has multiple complex functions that these devices are unable to accomplish.[21,48]

Molecular Adsorbent Recirculating System

Molecular adsorbent recirculating system (MARS) is a hemodialysis unit used to perform albumin dialysis that uses an additional dialysate circuit, which contains albumin-bound membrane to clean and recirculate the albumin. Albumin dialysis aids in the removal of both protein-bound and water-soluble substances via diffusion across the membrane due to the excess albumin in the dialysate.[49]

The MARS has been used in the last decade for the removal of toxic metabolites that accumulate in FHF. MARS is an extracorporeal hepatic assistance technique, which is well tolerated and can be used repeatedly over prolonged periods of time. MARS enables the removal of water-soluble and -insoluble, albumin-bound toxic molecules that can accumulate in the blood of patients with FHF.[49] By reducing the ammonia levels along with excretion and elimination of free fatty acids and aromatic amino acids, it is hoped that it could reduce HE, CE, and ICP and be a bridging device to liver transplantation in patients with FHF.[49,50] A randomized controlled trial of 102 patients with FHF, however, was unable to provide definitive efficacy or safety conclusions, because many patients had a liver transplant before administration of MARS.[51]

Bioartificial Liver Systems

Bioartifical liver (BAL) systems use human or nonhuman liver cells for detoxification and secretion of hepatocyte-derived factors. These systems serve as both excretory and synthetic substitutes of liver function.[49] BAL systems have demonstrated some improvement in encephalopathy.[21] The largest prospective, randomized, multicenter controlled trial of 171 patients with FHF failed, however, to show survival significance at 30 days.[52] In addition, because these systems use nonhuman hepatocytes or hepatoblastoma cell lines, there is concern that these systems can cause zoonosis, cancer, and new antibodies.[50]

SUMMARY

HE development in FHF is associated with decrease in survival rates. CE and ICH are secondary to elevated ammonia levels and are responsible for death in patients with FHF. Infection and the resulting inflammation can cause further worsening of HE in FHF patients. Ruling out other causes of altered mental status, identifying and correcting the precipitants, and treatment should all be started simultaneously. Liver transplant evaluation should be considered in all patients who present with HE and FHF. The utility of lactulose and rifaximin for treating encephalopathy in FHF is unclear. N-acetylcysteine can be used for both acetaminophen- and nonacetaminophen-induced FHF.

REFERENCES

1. Vilstrup H, Amodio P, Bajaj J, et al. Hepatic encephalopathy in chronic liver disease: 2014 Practice Guideline by the American Association for the Study of Liver Diseases and the European Association for the Study of the Liver. Hepatology 2014;60:715–35.
2. Wang DW, Yin YM, Yao YM. Advances in the management of acute liver failure. World J Gastroenterol 2013;19:7069–77.
3. Bjerring PN, Eefsen M, Hansen BA, et al. The brain in acute liver failure. A tortuous path from hyperammonemia to cerebral edema. Metab Brain Dis 2009;24:5–14.
4. Vaquero J, Chung C, Cahill ME, et al. Pathogenesis of hepatic encephalopathy in acute liver failure. Semin Liver Dis 2003;23:259–69.
5. American Association for the Study of Liver Diseases, European Association for the Study of the Liver. Hepatic encephalopathy in chronic liver disease: 2014 practice guideline by the European Association for the Study of the Liver and the American Association for the Study of Liver Diseases. J Hepatol 2014;61: 642–59.
6. Detry O, De Roover A, Honore P, et al. Brain edema and intracranial hypertension in fulminant hepatic failure: pathophysiology and management. World J Gastroenterol 2006;12:7405–12.
7. Lee WM. Acute liver failure. Semin Respir Crit Care Med 2012;33:36–45.
8. Mukherjee KK, Chhabra R, Khosla VK. Raised intracranial pressure in hepatic encephalopathy. Indian J Gastroenterol 2003;22(Suppl 2):S62–5.
9. O'Grady JG, Schalm SW, Williams R. Acute liver failure: redefining the syndromes. Lancet 1993;342:273–5.

10. Vaquero J, Polson J, Chung C, et al. Infection and the progression of hepatic encephalopathy in acute liver failure. Gastroenterology 2003;125: 755–64.
11. Prakash R, Mullen KD. Mechanisms, diagnosis and management of hepatic encephalopathy. Nat Rev Gastroenterol Hepatol 2010;7:515–25.
12. Mohsenin V. Assessment and management of cerebral edema and intracranial hypertension in acute liver failure. J Crit Care 2013;28:783–91.
13. Hassanein T, Blei AT, Perry W, et al. Performance of the hepatic encephalopathy scoring algorithm in a clinical trial of patients with cirrhosis and severe hepatic encephalopathy. Am J Gastroenterol 2009;104:1392–400.
14. Ferenci P, Lockwood A, Mullen K, et al. Hepatic encephalopathy–definition, nomenclature, diagnosis, and quantification: final report of the working party at the 11th World Congresses of Gastroenterology, Vienna, 1998. Hepatology 2002;35:716–21.
15. Clemmesen JO, Larsen FS, Kondrup J, et al. Cerebral herniation in patients with acute liver failure is correlated with arterial ammonia concentration. Hepatology 1999;29:648–53.
16. Rovira A, Alonso J, Cordoba J. MR imaging findings in hepatic encephalopathy. AJNR Am J Neuroradiol 2008;29:1612–21.
17. Kim YK, Seo H, Yu J, et al. Noninvasive estimation of raised intracranial pressure using ocular ultrasonography in liver transplant recipients with acute liver failure -A report of two cases. Korean J Anesthesiol 2013;64:451–5.
18. Soldatos T, Chatzimichail K, Papathanasiou M, et al. Optic nerve sonography: a new window for the non-invasive evaluation of intracranial pressure in brain injury. Emerg Med J 2009;26:630–4.
19. Moretti R, Pizzi B, Cassini F, et al. Reliability of optic nerve ultrasound for the evaluation of patients with spontaneous intracranial hemorrhage. Neurocrit Care 2009;11:406–10.
20. Lee WM. Drug-induced acute liver failure. Clin Liver Dis 2013;17:575–86, viii.
21. Lee WM, Stravitz RT, Larson AM. Introduction to the revised American Association for the Study of Liver Diseases Position Paper on acute liver failure 2011. Hepatology 2012;55:965–7.
22. Albrecht J, Norenberg MD. Glutamine: a Trojan horse in ammonia neurotoxicity. Hepatology 2006;44:788–94.
23. Bernardi P, Krauskopf A, Basso E, et al. The mitochondrial permeability transition from in vitro artifact to disease target. FEBS J 2006;273:2077–99.
24. Cordoba J, Sanpedro F, Alonso J, et al. 1H magnetic resonance in the study of hepatic encephalopathy in humans. Metab Brain Dis 2002;17:415–29.
25. Rolando N, Wade J, Davalos M, et al. The systemic inflammatory response syndrome in acute liver failure. Hepatology 2000;32:734–9.
26. Karvellas CJ, Cavazos J, Battenhouse H, et al. Effects of antimicrobial prophylaxis and blood stream infections in patients with acute liver failure: a retrospective cohort study. Clin Gastroenterol Hepatol 2014;12(11):1942–9.e1.
27. Sales I, Dzierba AL, Smithburger PL, et al. Use of acetylcysteine for non-acetaminophen-induced acute liver failure. Ann Hepatol 2013;12:6–10.
28. Bajaj JS. Management options for minimal hepatic encephalopathy. Expert Rev Gastroenterol Hepatol 2008;2:785–90.
29. van Leeuwen PA, van Berlo CL, Soeters PB. New mode of action for lactulose. Lancet 1988;1:55–6.
30. Mullen KD, Amodio P, Morgan MY. Therapeutic studies in hepatic encephalopathy. Metab Brain Dis 2007;22:407–23.

31. Stravitz RT, Kramer AH, Davern T, et al. Intensive care of patients with acute liver failure: recommendations of the U.S. Acute Liver Failure Study Group. Crit Care Med 2007;35:2498–508.
32. Polson J, Lee WM. AASLD position paper: the management of acute liver failure. Hepatology 2005;41:1179–97.
33. Conn HO, Leevy CM, Vlahcevic ZR, et al. Comparison of lactulose and neomycin in the treatment of chronic portal-systemic encephalopathy. A double blind controlled trial. Gastroenterology 1977;72:573–83.
34. Vaquero J, Fontana RJ, Larson AM, et al. Complications and use of intracranial pressure monitoring in patients with acute liver failure and severe encephalopathy. Liver Transpl 2005;11:1581–9.
35. Bass NM, Mullen KD, Sanyal A, et al. Rifaximin treatment in hepatic encephalopathy. N Engl J Med 2010;362:1071–81.
36. Plauth M. Nutrition and liver failure. Med Klin Intensivmed Notfmed 2013;108: 391–5 [in German].
37. Plauth M, Cabre E, Campillo B, et al. ESPEN Guidelines on parenteral nutrition: hepatology. Clin Nutr 2009;28:436–44.
38. Als-Nielsen B, Koretz RL, Kjaergard LL, et al. Branched-chain amino acids for hepatic encephalopathy. Cochrane Database Syst Rev 2003;(2):CD001939.
39. Mas A. Hepatic encephalopathy: from pathophysiology to treatment. Digestion 2006;73(Suppl 1):86–93.
40. Frontera JA, Kalb T. Neurological management of fulminant hepatic failure. Neurocrit Care 2011;14:318–27.
41. Krishnamoorthy V, Beckmann K, Mueller M, et al. Perioperative estimation of the intracranial pressure using the optic nerve sheath diameter during liver transplantation. Liver Transpl 2013;19:246–9.
42. Singh RK, Poddar B, Singhal S, et al. Continuous hypertonic saline for acute liver failure. Indian J Gastroenterol 2011;30:178–80.
43. Larsen FS, Bjerring PN. Acute liver failure. Curr Opin Crit Care 2011;17:160–4.
44. Jalan R. Intracranial hypertension in acute liver failure: pathophysiological basis of rational management. Semin Liver Dis 2003;23:271–82.
45. Rabinstein AA. Treatment of brain edema in acute liver failure. Curr Treat Options Neurol 2010;12:129–41.
46. Geurts M, Macleod MR, Kollmar R, et al. Therapeutic hypothermia and the risk of infection: a systematic review and meta-analysis. Crit Care Med 2014;42:231–42.
47. Strauss GI. The effect of hyperventilation upon cerebral blood flow and metabolism in patients with fulminant hepatic failure. Dan Med Bull 2007;54:99–111.
48. Rademacher S, Oppert M, Jorres A. Artificial extracorporeal liver support therapy in patients with severe liver failure. Expert Rev Gastroenterol Hepatol 2011;5: 591–9.
49. Tan HK. Molecular adsorbent recirculating system (MARS). Ann Acad Med Singapore 2004;33:329–35.
50. Novelli G, Rossi M, Pretagostini R, et al. MARS (Molecular Adsorbent Recirculating System): experience in 34 cases of acute liver failure. Liver 2002;22(Suppl 2): 43–7.
51. Saliba F, Camus C, Durand F, et al. Albumin dialysis with a noncell artificial liver support device in patients with acute liver failure: a randomized, controlled trial. Ann Intern Med 2013;159:522–31.
52. Demetriou AA, Brown RS Jr, Busuttil RW, et al. Prospective, randomized, multicenter, controlled trial of a bioartificial liver in treating acute liver failure. Ann Surg 2004;239:660–7 [discussion: 667–70].

Legal Responsibilities of Physicians When They Diagnose Hepatic Encephalopathy

CrossMark

John M. Vierling, MD

KEYWORDS

- Cirrhosis • Portal hypertension • Hepatic encephalopathy
- Covert hepatic encephalopathy • Overt hepatic encephalopathy • Cognition
- Motor function • Legal affairs

KEY POINTS

- Covert hepatic encephalopathy (CHE) and overt hepatic encephalopathy impair the ability to drive or operate machinery.
- CHE has no clinical manifestations, and can be diagnosed only from specialized tests; however, no consensus exists regarding which tests to use.
- At present, physicians in the United States have no medical legal responsibility to perform tests to detect CHE.
- Physicians must know and abide by their state-specific reporting laws for impairment and know the legal ramifications of reporting or not reporting.
- Mandatory or permissive reporting by physicians does not violate physician-patient confidentiality statutes or the protected health information statutes of the Health Insurance Portability and Accountability Act.

INTRODUCTION

Hepatic encephalopathy (HE) is a spectrum of neuropsychiatric abnormalities observed in patients with either acute or chronic liver dysfunction and portal-systemic shunting (**Fig. 1**).[1] It is most commonly observed in patients with cirrhosis of the liver. The neuropsychiatric spectrum of abnormalities can also occur in patients without liver disease; thus, the diagnosis of HE requires exclusion of other central nervous system diseases. In cirrhotic patients, HE can be either covert (previously designated as minimal or subclinical HE) or overt. At present, covert HE (CHE) can be diagnosed only with specialized neurocognitive testing.[1–3] CHE is a major risk factor

Disclosure: Dr. Vierling is a Scientific Advisory Board Consultant for Salix and Hyperion. He has also received research grant funding from Hyperion.
Departments of Medicine and Surgery, Baylor St Luke's Liver Center, Baylor College of Medicine, 6620 Main Street, Suite 1425, Houston, TX 77030, USA
E-mail address: vierling@bcm.edu

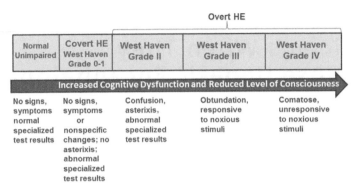

Fig. 1. Classification and spectrum of covert and overt HE.

for development of overt HE (OHE),[1,2] characterized by detectable alterations of mood, behavior, and personality, confusion, inability to concentrate, and decreased cognition.[1] OHE is also associated with movement disorders, including hypertonus and asterixis. As OHE progresses in grade, patients become stuporous and ultimately comatose (see **Fig. 1**).

CHE is a vexing clinical problem because of the absence of clinically evident cognitive or neurologic symptoms.[1,2] The diagnosis of CHE requires sensitive neuropsychological cognitive testing. However, no agreement exists among experts about which standardized screening tools should be used to diagnose CHE.[4] Studies using a variety of such tests have concluded that the prevalence of CHE in cirrhotic patients ranges from 30% to 80%.[2]

Numerous studies indicate that cirrhotic patients with CHE may have significantly reduced fitness to operate motor vehicles or safely perform in occupations requiring concentration, dexterity, and normal reaction times for safe performance.[2,5] Patients with OHE have demonstrable impairments of driving skills (discussed later). Successful medical therapy alleviates the cognitive and neurologic symptoms of OHE, returning treated patients with OHE to a cognitive state of CHE.[6] Medical therapy for patients with CHE may improve driving impairment.[7]

Physicians caring for patients with either CHE or OHE have had scant guidance regarding their legal responsibilities for reporting such patients as potentially unsafe drivers to their state's departments of motor vehicles.[8,9] In the absence of specific guidance, potential liability exists for both the patient and physician. Although medical malpractice lawsuits have been brought against physicians for motor vehicle accidents (MVAs) caused by impaired patients without liver diseases, to date, no publications report lawsuits against physicians caring for cirrhotic patients with either CHE or OHE.

The goals of this article are 4-fold:

- First, to describe the nature and the frequency of the impairment of patients with CHE and OHE.
- Second, to review the policies for reporting impaired drivers in the 50 states of the United States.
- Third, to review the current status of legal responsibilities of physicians diagnosing and caring for cirrhotic patients with CHE or OHE.
- Fourth, to provide evidence-based recommendations for identification, counseling, and reporting of impaired patients with CHE or OHE.

EVIDENCE THAT COVERT HEPATIC ENCEPHALOPATHY IMPAIRS SKILLS NECESSARY FOR SAFE DRIVING OR OPERATING MACHINERY

In 1986, Gitlin and colleagues[10] described the syndrome of CHE in patients with histologically proven cirrhosis who otherwise appeared healthy and had not undergone surgical shunt procedures. All 37 patients had normal mental status examinations and neurologic examinations, and their cirrhosis was considered clinically well compensated. None required dietary restrictions or medications. Most continued to operate motor vehicles. Psychometric testing was performed in these patients as well as in a control group of 19 patients with a history of alcoholism or other medical disorders in the absence of clinical or biochemical evidence of cirrhosis. Patients and controls were matched by age, sex, level of education, and alcohol consumption. Testing included an electroencephalogram (EEG), fasting arterial NH_3, liver enzymes and total bilirubin, and a battery of verbal and performance-based psychometric tests. Among the 37 cirrhotic patients, the EEG was abnormal in 3 (8.3%) and the fasting arterial NH_3 level was increased in 17 (45.9%). Among the 37 patients, 26 (70.3%) failed 2 or more of the psychometric tests, compared with only 2 (10.5%) of the controls. The investigators concluded that 70% of their cirrhotic patients had CHE and that the principal impairment was in performance tests, not verbal skills tests. They expressed concern about the consequences of impaired performance, especially in occupations requiring the use of mechanical devices or skilled behaviors.

In 1996, Eisenburg[11] concluded that the neuropsychiatric impairment of CHE was expressed in everyday life by "impairment of driving ability, and at work by impaired ability to operate a machine." He further concluded that lowering of blood NH_3 levels using lactulose or ornithine-aspartate improved CHE.

In 2004, Wein and colleagues[12] reported driving impairment of patients with cirrhosis and CHE. The diagnosis of CHE was made using 3 psychometric tests (number connection tests part A, digit symbol tests, and complex choice reaction tests). Subjects performed a standardized driving test over a 35-km (22-miles) course for a duration of 90 minutes, accompanied by a professional driving instructor who was blinded to the subject's diagnosis and test results. The driving assessment included 4 global driving categories (car handling, adaptation to traffic situations, caution, and maneuvering) and 17 specific driving actions, such as changing lanes, and overtaking and passing vehicles. Among 274 consecutive patients with cirrhosis of the liver, 48 (17.5%) fulfilled medical and driving performance criteria for inclusion: 34 had no evidence of CHE, whereas 14 met criteria for CHE. The control group consisted of 49 subjects in a stable phase of chronic gastroenterological disease with normal liver enzymes and bilirubin. Patients with CHE showed a significant reduction in driving scores compared with either cirrhotic patients without CHE or with controls ($P<.05$). Statistically significant differences in specific driving actions included the need for the instructor to intervene in 5 of the 14 subjects with CHE to avoid an accident. The results indicated that the ability to drive a car for 35 km over a 90-minute period while observed by a professional instructor was significantly impaired in cirrhotic patients with CHE but unimpaired in cirrhotic patients without CHE. The investigators concluded that patients with cirrhosis should be tested for CHE, and, if diagnosed, informed of the risk of driving and treated to improve their psychometric test results. These results differed from those of a prior driving study of 30 minutes' duration that failed to identify impaired driving skills in cirrhotics with CHE.

In 2008, Bajaj and colleagues[13] reported impairment of simulated navigational skills in cirrhotic patients with CHE. Navigation constitutes a complex task, requiring functions of memory and other psychomotor domains adversely affected by CHE. The study population included 49 patients with nonalcoholic cirrhosis who underwent psychometric testing using tests of block design, digit symbol, and number connection test A. Based on these tests, 34 of the 49 (69%) had CHE and 15 (31%) did not. The control group consisted of 48 healthy persons matched for age and education. All cirrhotic subjects and control subjects underwent a battery of psychometric tests, an inhibitory control test, and a driving simulation test. The driving simulation study was conducted in 4 parts. The first consisted of training, the second consisted of driving with negative outcomes representing MVAs, the third consisted of assessment of divided attention, and the fourth assessed navigational ability by driving along a marked path on a map. Navigational ability was significantly impaired in cirrhotic subjects with CHE ($P = .007$). Subjects with CHE scored less well in divided attention tasks than cirrhotics without CHE or controls ($P = .001$). Subjects with CHE had a higher rate of accidents during simulated driving compared with either cirrhotics without CHE or controls ($P = .004$). The frequencies of accidents and illegal turns were significantly correlated ($r = 0.51$; $P = .001$). Impaired inhibitory control testing correlated with both illegal turns ($r = 0.6$) and accidents ($r = 0.44$). The investigators concluded that cirrhotic subjects with CHE had markedly impaired navigation skills caused by deficits in response inhibition and attention.

Bajaj and colleagues[14] next investigated the insight of patients with CHE regarding their impaired driving skills using the driving behavior survey (DBS), a validated questionnaire that contains a driving skills section that assesses attention. The DBS can be either self-administered or administered by an observer. The patient's self-assessment using the DBS was compared with that of an observer who assessed their driving skills in a driving simulator of navigation and simple driving tasks. In addition, an adult familiar with the subjects' driving history independently completed the DBS. Among 47 cirrhotic patients, 36 met criteria for CHE and 11 did not. The CHE group had a significantly higher number of simulator crashes ($P = .001$) and higher rates of illegal turns ($P = .0001$) than either cirrhotics without CHE or controls. Despite their impaired performance, cirrhotics with CHE scored their own driving skills as being comparable with the self-assessments of cirrhotics without CHE or controls. In contrast, independent observers rated cirrhotics with CHE, both in total score and driving skills, at a much lower level than their self-assessments or observer assessments of cirrhotics without CHE or controls ($P = .0001$). Self-assessments of cirrhotics without CHE and controls were similar to the ratings of the independent observers. The investigators concluded that cirrhotic subjects with CHE lacked awareness of their impaired driving skills, assessing them as normal. Thus, cirrhotic patients with CHE are unlikely to provide an accurate description of their driving skills when questioned by health care providers.

Bajaj and colleagues[15] validated the research test results of impaired driving by showing that patients with CHE also had excessive MVAs and traffic violations. They reviewed self-reporting and Department of Transportation (DOT) records of MVAs and traffic violations over the preceding year. Patients were then followed prospectively for a year to determine rates of MVAs or traffic violations. MVAs in the prior year occurred exclusively in cirrhotics with CHE (17%; $P = .0004$). Patients with CHE had significantly higher rates of traffic violations (17%) compared with cirrhotics without CHE (3%; relative risk = 5.77; $P = .004$). Cirrhotics with CHE had significantly higher rates of MVAs over the next year compared with those without CHE (22% vs 7%; odds ratio = 4.51; $P = .03$). There was excellent agreement between self-reported events and the official reports.

CLINICAL TESTING FOR COVERT HEPATIC ENCEPHALOPATHY

The most vexing problem is the lack of a validated test or tests to accurately define the presence or absence of CHE.[3,5] As noted earlier, a variety of tests were performed to categorize cirrhotic subjects into groups with and without CHE. The battery of tests used to conduct current research in CHE cannot readily be used (or readily afforded) in clinical practice. Recent studies indicated that interindividual and intraindividual variability significantly affects cognitive performance in several neuropsychological diseases.

Clarification of the types and magnitude of impairment associated with CHE depends on the accuracy of the diagnosis of CHE. Among the methods used to establish the diagnosis of CHE are standardized psychometric batteries, neuropsychological testing, computerized testing, and comprehensive neuropsychological examinations.[3] Several of these tests are copyrighted and require a specific psychological or neurologic expertise for access, administration, and interpretation. As a result, most hepatologists responding to an American Association for the Study of Liver Diseases survey noted an inability to test cirrhotic patients for CHE.[16] A more recent international survey indicated marked geographic differences in the preference for specific tests for CHE.[4] The details of available tests and their correlations with driving impairment are beyond the scope of this article but are discussed by Flamm elsewhere in this issue.

CAN TREATMENT OF COVERT HEPATIC ENCEPHALOPATHY PREVENT MOTOR VEHICLE ACCIDENTS?

In the United States, the annual cost of MVAs has been estimated to be more than $200 billion. The societal costs are severe, including unnecessary death, treatment of traumatic injuries, motor vehicle damage, loss of work and family-related productivity, uninsured cost to employers, and administrative cost. Several studies indicate that medical treatment can improve or reverse CHE; however, the specific tests used to define CHE have varied. Lactulose therapy has been tested in patients with CHE and shown to reverse the performance deficits on psychometric tests used to define CHE.[17] The applicability of lactulose treatment is reduced by problematic adherence in response to bloating and diarrhea associated with its use. Rifaximin has also been used for the treatment of patients with CHE and improved performance on driving simulator tests in a randomized, placebo-controlled trial.[7]

Bajaj and colleagues[18] conducted a cost-effectiveness analysis of the benefits of various strategies to diagnose and treat CHE and reduce MVA-related costs. They compared 5 management strategies for CHE:

1. Treatment of all cirrhotics
2. Diagnosis by neuropsychological examination followed by treatment
3. Diagnosis by standard psychometric tests followed by treatment
4. Diagnosis by rapid screening using inhibitory control tests followed by treatment
5. No diagnostic testing for CHE or treatment

Only lactulose or rifaximin were considered as treatments and were assumed able to reduce MVA rates to those of age-matched noncirrhotics following adjustment of beneficial effects for treatment compliance. Their analysis used a Markov model of a simulated cohort of 1000 cirrhotic patients without overt HE from entry through development of CHE and later overt HE with a 5-year follow-up, which included biannual testing for CHE. All 4 treatment strategies were cost-effective compared with the status quo of not diagnosing or treating CHE. The alternative strategies also cost less per year than the estimated $42,100 societal cost of a single MVA. As expected, lactulose therapy was significantly less expensive than rifaximin therapy. Rifaximin therapy was not cost saving at its current price, but would be if the monthly cost were less than $353. The model estimated savings of $1.7 million to $3.6 million over a 5-year period with the variation depending on the strategy used for diagnosis and treatment.

The encouraging data on the effectiveness of treatment of patients with CHE in its potential impact in reducing MVAs underscores the urgency of identifying and implementing use of evidence-based diagnostic criteria for CHE. Based on the evidence that currently available therapies may reverse CHE, randomized controlled trials of the use of therapy to retard or prevent development of CHE are also a high priority. If development of CHE could be prevented, it might also significantly reduce progression to OHE, because CHE is its predominant risk factor.[1]

LEGAL RAMIFICATIONS FOR PHYSICIANS WHO DIAGNOSE AND TREAT PATIENTS WITH HEPATIC ENCEPHALOPATHY

In 2011, Cohen and colleagues[9] evaluated the legal ramifications for physicians treating patients with HE who drive. They examined the motor vehicle code of each state and the requirements for physician reporting of potentially impaired patients with CHE or OHE. They also searched for lawsuits against physicians related to MVAs involving patients with HE. In addition, they looked for lawsuits against patients with HE involved in MVAs. States with statutes requiring reporting can be divided into mandatory reporting states and permissive reporting states. The laws of mandatory reporting states required a physician to report potentially impaired drivers or contained mention of fines or criminal penalties for physicians who did not report such a driver. In contrast, permissive reporting states had statutes allowing a physician to report an impaired driver without mandating such reporting.

The Department of Motor Vehicle codes regarding medically impaired drivers varied considerably among states. The definition of a medically impaired driver also varied, ranging from specific mention of a seizure disorder and generalized terms that included "lapses in consciousness," "neuropsychiatric conditions," and "cognitive impairment." None of the DOT codes specifically mentioned HE or cognitive impairment or neuropsychiatric conditions of advanced liver disease or cirrhosis.

Table 1 summarizes the similarities and differences among the 50 states with respect to laws regarding physicians' responsibility to report medically impaired drivers and laws allowing concerned citizens to report drivers suspected of impairment. For this review, an extensive Internet-based search of current DOT requirements in 50 states was conducted to update information presented by Cohen and colleagues.[9] All states require applicants for driver's licenses to answer health-related questions before being issued a new license or renewing an existing one. Despite the requirement of self-reporting of health status by applicants for a license, only a few states have explicit provisions for dealing with persons who have developed medical conditions that could impair their ability to drive safely.

At present, physicians are mandated to report medically impaired drivers in only 8 of 50 states (16%). **Table 2** summarizes the categories of reportable neuropsychiatric impairments. States requiring mandatory reporting by physicians provided legal immunity to the physician. Permissive reporting statutes exist in 33 states (66%); the remaining 9 states (18%) have no specific reporting statutes. Among the 33 states with permissive reporting statutes, 24 (73%) provide legal immunity to the reporting physician, whereas 9 (31%) do not. Legal immunity is provided by the 3 states with statutes allowing reports by concerned citizens. In the 9 states without specific reporting statutes, 1 (11%) provided immunity to a reporting physician and 8 (89%) did not.

The laws in these states varied as to whether physicians bore liability for not reporting a patient who subsequently was involved in an MVA (discussed later). In 38 (76%) states, a medical advisory board was empowered to work with the DOT. There was great variation among states with respect to the medical advisory board's responsibilities and authority.

Patient-Physician Confidentiality Issues

Many legal circumstances exist in which the obligation of physicians to maintain patient confidentiality is subordinate to a duty to protect persons from harm. Common examples include reporting child abuse, sexual abuse, gunshot wounds, viral hepatitis, and sexually transmitted diseases. The American Medical Association's statement of ethics provides that, "A physician may not reveal the confidence entrusted to him in the course of medical attendance, or the deficiencies he may observe in the character of patients, unless he is required to do so by law or unless it becomes necessary in order to protect the welfare of the individual or of the community." The American Medical Association believes that, "reporting of impaired patients to departments of transportation should be a matter of professional judgment, undertaken after discussion between physicians and their patients."[19] Mandatory reporting laws of several states are consistent with these statements.

Confidentiality of Protected Health Information

The Health Insurance Portability and Accountability Act (HIPPA) does not restrict medical professionals from disclosing a patient's protected health information when disclosure to a state agency is required by law.[20] Therefore, HIPPA regulations do not apply to physicians who comply with mandatory reporting laws, and no individual consent to release protected health information is required.

Most, but not all, of the states with permissive reporting laws provide strict confidentiality for physician reports and legal immunity for reporting. In states not providing immunity, it is unclear whether a physician could be held liable for providing protected health information without a patient's consent under HIPPA. Physicians in these states should seek legal guidance to answer this question.

Liabilities for Reporting or not Reporting an Impaired Patient

All but 1 of the states with mandatory reporting statutes provides legal immunity. Pennsylvania, a mandatory reporting state, addresses this frequently asked question by stating that, "If you DO report, you are immune from any civil or criminal liability. No action may be brought against any person or agency for providing the required information; however, if you DO NOT report, there is a possibility that you could be held responsible as a proximate cause of an accident resulting in death, injury or property loss caused by your patient. Also, providers who do not comply with their legal requirement to report may be convicted of a summary criminal offense."[21]

Lawsuits

Cohen and colleagues[9] examined legal databases, law journals, and law reviews in both federal and state courts, querying the following medical terms: cirrhosis, end-stage liver disease, encephalopathy, HE, liver coma, or liver confusion. These medical terms were matched against all terms related to MVA, including car, automobile, truck, vehicle, auto, or accident. Their search identified 176 cases matching at least 1 of the medical terms plus 1 of the accident-related terms.

None of the cases involved litigation for the failure of a physician to admonish a patient not to drive or failure to diagnose HE in a patient who subsequently had an MVA.

Table 1
Reporting requirements for medically impaired drivers 2015

State	Medical Advisory Board	Physician Reporting Requirements for Cognitive Impairment			Legal Immunity	Citizen Reporting of Suspected Impaired Drivers	Impairment Laws for Drugs and Alcohol		DEC/DRE Law Enforcement Training[c]
		Mandatory	Permissive	None			Per Se Drug Laws[b]	Alcohol	
Alabama	Yes	—	Yes	—	Yes	—	—	Yes	Yes
Alaska	No	—	—	Yes	No	—	—	Yes	Yes
Arizona	Yes	—	Yes	—	Yes	—	Yes	Yes	Yes
Arkansas	No	—	Yes	—	No	—	—	Yes	Yes
California	Yes	Yes	—	—	Yes	—	—	Yes	Yes
Colorado	No	—	Yes	—	Yes	—	—	Yes	Yes
Connecticut	Yes	—	Yes	—	Yes	—	—	Yes	Yes
Delaware	Yes	Yes	—	—	Yes	—	Yes	Yes	Yes
Florida	Yes	—	Yes	—	Yes	Yes[a]	—	Yes	Yes
Georgia	Yes	Yes	—	—	No	—	Yes	Yes	Yes
Hawaii	No	—	—	Yes	No	—	—	Yes	Yes
Idaho	No	—	Yes	—	No	—	—	Yes	Yes
Illinois	Yes	—	Yes	—	Yes	—	Yes	Yes	Yes
Indiana	Yes	—	Yes	—	Yes	—	Yes	Yes	Yes
Iowa	Yes	—	Yes	—	Yes	—	Yes	Yes	Yes
Kansas	Yes	—	Yes	—	Yes	—	—	Yes	Yes
Kentucky	Yes	—	Yes	—	Yes	—	Yes	Yes	Yes
Louisiana	Yes	—	Yes	—	Yes	—	—	Yes	Yes
Maine	Yes	Yes	—	—	Yes	Yes[a]	—	Yes	Yes
Maryland	Yes	—	Yes	—	Yes	—	—	Yes	Yes
Massachusetts	Yes	—	—	Yes	No	—	—	Yes	Yes
Michigan	Yes	—	Yes	—	No	—	Yes	Yes	Yes
Minnesota	Yes	—	Yes	—	Yes	—	Yes	Yes	Yes
Mississippi	Yes	—	—	Yes	No	—	Yes	Yes	Yes
Missouri	Yes	—	Yes	—	Yes	Yes[a]	—	Yes	Yes

Montana	No	—	—	—	Yes	—	—	Yes	Yes
Nebraska	Yes	—	Yes	—	No	—	—	Yes	Yes
Nevada	Yes	Yes	—	—	Yes	—	Yes	Yes	Yes
New Hampshire	No	—	Yes	—	No	—	—	Yes	Yes
New Jersey	Yes	Yes	—	—	Yes	—	—	Yes	Yes
New Mexico	Yes	—	Yes	—	Yes	—	—	Yes	Yes
New York	Yes	—	Yes	—	No	—	—	Yes	Yes
North Carolina	Yes	—	Yes	—	Yes	—	Yes	Yes	Yes
North Dakota	Yes	—	Yes	—	Yes	—	—	Yes	Yes
Ohio	No	—	Yes	—	No	—	Yes	Yes	Yes
Oklahoma	Yes	—	Yes	—	Yes	—	—	Yes	Yes
Oregon	No	Yes	—	—	Yes	—	—	Yes	Yes
Pennsylvania	Yes	Yes	—	—	Yes	—	Yes	Yes	Yes
Rhode Island	Yes	—	Yes	—	Yes	—	Yes	Yes	Yes
South Carolina	Yes	—	—	Yes	No	—	—	Yes	Yes
South Dakota	Yes	—	Yes	—	No	—	—	Yes	Yes
Tennessee	Yes	—	—	Yes	Yes	—	—	Yes	Yes
Texas	Yes	—	Yes	—	Yes	—	—	Yes	Yes
Utah	Yes	—	Yes	—	Yes	—	Yes	Yes	Yes
Vermont	No	—	—	Yes	No	—	—	Yes	Yes
Virginia	Yes	—	Yes	—	No	—	Yes	Yes	Yes
Washington	No	—	—	Yes	No	—	Yes	Yes	Yes
West Virginia	Yes	—	Yes	—	No	—	—	Yes	Yes
Wisconsin	Yes	—	Yes	—	Yes	—	Yes	Yes	Yes
Wyoming	No	—	—	Yes	No	—	—	Yes	Yes
Total States	—	8	33	9	32	3	19	50	50

Abbreviations: DEC, drug evaluation and classification programs; DRE, drug recognition expert.
[a] Immunity extended to citizens who report potentially impaired drivers.
[b] Per se drug laws forbid any presence of a prohibited substance or drug in the driver's body while in control of the vehicle, without any other evidence of impairment.
[c] DECs that train law enforcement officers to become certified DREs.

Table 2
Categories of impairments affecting safe driving to be considered by physicians

Neurologic Impairments, Primary Diseases, and Cerebrovascular Accident	Cognitive Impairments	Conditions Affecting Awareness and Driving Safety	Drugs and Alcohol
Ataxia or balance dysfunction	Visual perception and attention dysfunction	Seizure disorders	Alcohol
Motor control impairments	Abnormal memory	Hypoglycemia	Marijuana
Vision dysfunctions	Executive functions disorder[a]	Syncope	Prescription medications[b]
	Coordination dysfunction	Cardiac diseases	Illicit medications[c]
		Neurologic diseases	
		Excessive daytime sleepiness	
		Sleep disorders	

[a] Working memory, inhibitory control, problem solving.
[b] Opiates, benzodiazepines, sleeping medications, antianxiety medications, and so forth.
[c] Heroin, cocaine, methamphetamine, and so forth.

Moreover, none of the cases involved litigation against a patient with HE for involvement in an MVA while driving.

An Internet search conducted for this review identified multiple plaintiff medical malpractice Web sites using the term encephalopathy. HE was occasionally listed among the encephalopathies. HE was not listed or discussed among the types of encephalopathies for which legal action could be brought for failure to diagnose or properly treat.

CURRENT PRACTICES REGARDING HEPATIC ENCEPHALOPATHY AND DRIVING

Lauridsen and Bajaj[4] recently summarized the results of a worldwide, systematic, electronic survey of clinical experts in HE regarding diagnosis, management, and the issue of driving in patients with CHE or OHE. The questionnaire was sent to 285 experts, and the response rate was 35%. Respondents were from 23 different countries: North and South America (n = 28), Europe (n = 48), and Asia (n = 21).

Ninety-nine percent of respondents agreed that CHE and OHE detrimentally affect driving skills. All respondents answered questions related to driving in the context of their local driving regulations. Only 20% of clinicians discussed driving with most of their patients with HE, asking more than 60% of patients about their driving history. In contrast, another 20% of clinicians asked less than 5% of their patients about driving.

Overall clinical impressions were most frequently used to determine whether drivers were unsafe. Other drivers were categorized as unsafe based on driving history (45%), psychomotor testing (40%), time since an episode of OHE (38%), or the opinions of caregivers (37%). At some point, most clinicians had urged patients not to drive: specifically, 79% of patients with an episode of OHE within 3 months and 67% of patients with CHE. Very few patients had been admonished not to drive in the month before completing the survey.

In the Americas, 86% of clinicians reported difficulty in dealing with driving issues related to HE. Although 98% think that both CHE and OHE impair driving skills, only 32% were aware of local driving laws regarding impairment. Only 29% obtained a driving history in most of their patients. Screening for CHE was offered by 54% of clinicians (preferred tests were quality-of-life questionnaire or Stroop test). Treatment of CHE was offered on a case-by-case basis by 65%. Treatment of CHE was never offered by 14% of clinicians, whereas 22% always offered treatment. These clinicians were willing to restrict driving for patients with a recent episode of OHE (79%), but less inclined to restrict driving in patients with controlled OHE (57%) or CHE (46%). However, these clinicians recommended driving restrictions at a much lower frequency: OHE episode within 3 months (21%), OHE currently controlled (0%), and CHE (7%). Only 21% used specialized tests for the purpose of identifying potentially unsafe drivers.

All respondents in the Americas thought that screening was important. Clinicians who did not perform screening cited multiple impediments: lack of time (78%), absence of consensus regarding what tests to use (54%), lack of adequate staffing (69%), and lack of consensus regarding consequences of screening (54%).

This survey reveals discrepancies between clinical opinions and clinical actions among experts in HE in the Americas. First, it is difficult to reconcile actions indicating that driving impairment is substantially different in patients whose OHE episode was controlled in the past 3 months versus patients with longer duration of medical control of OHE. The pathophysiology of HE indicates that control of OHE reverts patients to a state of CHE with persistent impairment (see **Fig. 1**). Second, the high degree of willingness to restrict driving in patients with CHE or OHE was not acted on. One of reasons may be the lack of awareness of applicable local laws regarding impaired driving. Another reason may relate to 86% of respondents finding it difficult to deal with issues of HE and driving. Although these difficulties included lack of time and staff, most respondents also cited lack of consensus about screening tests and the consequences of screening.

RECOMMENDATIONS

Box 1 lists the author's recommendations based on professional, moral, and ethical considerations of the published data. These recommendations are solely the view of the author and should not be construed as explicit guidance.

Box 1
Recommendations for physicians dealing with patients with CHE and OHE

Recognize that both CHE and OHE impair the ability to drive or operate machinery.

Know and abide by your state-specific reporting laws for impairment.

Know the legal ramifications of reporting and not reporting impairment in your state.

Recognize that CHE has no clinical manifestations and requires neurocognitive testing for diagnosis.

In the absence of validated diagnostic criteria for practitioners, physicians have no medical legal responsibility to perform diagnostic tests for CHE.

Mandatory and permissive reporting do not violate physician-patient confidentiality statures or the protected health information statutes of the HIPPA.

To date, no publications describe lawsuits against physicians caring for cirrhotic patients with either CHE or OHE.

Inform patients with CHE or OHE about the risks of driving or operating machinery.

Recommend a formal, professional driving assessment by the Department of Transportation for patients with CHE or OHE.

Recognize that only the state has the authority to determine who can or cannot drive.

SUMMARY

The legal responsibilities of physicians when they diagnose a patient with OHE vary among states (see **Table 1**). Thus, it is imperative that physicians know and abide by the explicit laws regarding reporting in their state and understand whether they have legal immunity for reporting. CHE and OHE impair the ability to drive or operate machinery. OHE represents a neuropsychiatric impairment that meets the general reporting criteria (see **Table 2**). At present, state medical advisory boards have not explicitly listed OHE as a reportable condition. Although published studies indicate that patients with CHE are also impaired, in the absence of validated guidelines for diagnostic testing, physicians in the United States have no medical legal requirement to perform tests to detect CHE. Physicians should advise patients with OHE about the risks of driving or operating machinery. Physicians should recommend that patients with either CHE or OHE have a professional driving evaluation conducted by the state's DOT. Only state agencies have the authority to determine who can or cannot drive. Mandatory or permissive reporting by physicians does not violate physician-patient confidentiality statutes or the protected health information statutes of the HIPPA. Although medical malpractice lawsuits have been brought against physicians for MVAs caused by impaired patients without liver diseases, to date, no publications describe lawsuits against physicians caring for cirrhotic patients with either CHE or OHE.

REFERENCES

1. Vilstrup H, Amodio P, Bajaj J, et al. Hepatic encephalopathy in chronic liver disease: 2014 practice guideline by the American Association for the Study of Liver Diseases and the European Association for the Study of the Liver. Hepatology 2014;60:715–35.
2. Stinton LM, Jayakumar S. Minimal hepatic encephalopathy. Can J Gastroenterol 2013;27:572–4.
3. Nabi E, Bajaj JS. Useful tests for hepatic encephalopathy in clinical practice. Curr Gastroenterol Rep 2014;16:362.
4. Lauridsen MM, Bajaj JS. Hepatic encephalopathy treatment and driving: a continental divide. J Hepatol 2015. [Epub ahead of print].
5. Kappus MR, Bajaj JS. Covert hepatic encephalopathy: not as minimal as you might think. Clin Gastroenterol Hepatol 2012;10:1208–19.
6. Bajaj JS, Schubert CM, Heuman DM, et al. Persistence of cognitive impairment after resolution of overt hepatic encephalopathy. Gastroenterology 2010;138:2332–40.
7. Bajaj JS, Heuman DM, Wade JB, et al. Rifaximin improves driving simulator performance in a randomized trial of patients with minimal hepatic encephalopathy. Gastroenterology 2011;140:478–87.
8. Berger JT, Rosner F, Kark P, et al. Reporting by physicians of impaired drivers and potentially impaired drivers. The Committee on Bioethical Issues of the Medical Society of the State of New York. J Gen Intern Med 2000;15:667–72.
9. Cohen SM, Kim A, Metropulos M, et al. Legal ramifications for physicians of patients who drive with hepatic encephalopathy. Clin Gastroenterol Hepatol 2011;9:156–60.
10. Gitlin N, Lewis DC, Hinkley L. The diagnosis and prevalence of subclinical hepatic encephalopathy in apparently healthy, ambulant, non-shunted patients with cirrhosis. J Hepatol 1986;3:75–82.

11. Eisenburg J. Hepatic minimal encephalopathy. The most frequently overlooked, clinically occult "metabolic syndrome" on the cirrhosis patient. Fortschr Med 1996;114:141–6 [in German].

12. Wein C, Koch H, Popp B, et al. Minimal hepatic encephalopathy impairs fitness to drive. Hepatology 2004;39:739–45.

13. Bajaj JS, Hafeezullah M, Hoffmann RG, et al. Navigation skill impairment: another dimension of the driving difficulties in minimal hepatic encephalopathy. Hepatology 2008;47:596–604.

14. Bajaj JS, Saeian K, Hafeezullah M, et al. Patients with minimal hepatic encephalopathy have poor insight into their driving skills. Clin Gastroenterol Hepatol 2008; 6:1135–9.

15. Bajaj JS, Saeian K, Schubert CM, et al. Minimal hepatic encephalopathy is associated with motor vehicle crashes: the reality beyond the driving test. Hepatology 2009;50:1175–83.

16. Bajaj JS, Etemadian A, Hafeezullah M, et al. Testing for minimal hepatic encephalopathy in the United States: an AASLD survey. Hepatology 2007;45:833–4.

17. Prasad S, Dhiman RK, Duseja A, et al. Lactulose improves cognitive functions and health-related quality of life in patients with cirrhosis who have minimal hepatic encephalopathy. Hepatology 2007;45:549–59.

18. Bajaj JS, Pinkerton SD, Sanyal AJ, et al. Diagnosis and treatment of minimal hepatic encephalopathy to prevent motor vehicle accidents: a cost-effectiveness analysis. Hepatology 2012;55:1164–71.

19. Available at: http://wwwama-assnorg/main/jsp/templates/primaryJSP/fullviewjsp?keyword=reporting+impaired+driver/. Accessed February 10, 2015.

20. Available at: http://www.hhsgov/ocr/hippa/. Accessed February 11, 2015.

21. Available at: http://www.pacode.com. Accessed February 11, 2015.

Printed and bound by CPI Group (UK) Ltd, Croydon, CR0 4YY

03/10/2024

01040496-0015